Healthcare Delivery in the U.S.A.

An Introduction

Endorsements for
Healthcare Delivery in the USA: An Introduction

By Margaret F. Schulte, PhD

"Margaret Schulte provides a concise introduction to the history, issues, terminology and structure of a very complex and often unwieldy industry—healthcare. This book would be helpful for those early in their careers or transitioning in from other industries to help improve quality and processes. I certainly wish I had this guide when I was starting in healthcare."

Mark Graban
Senior Lean Consultant
ValuMetrix Services
Ortho Clinical Diagnostics, Inc.
Author of *Lean Hospitals*

"Because traditional approaches to health reform aren't working, the business of medical care obviously needs new thinking from skilled professionals who can approach it from fresh perspectives. Many creative problem solvers from other industries would surely relish the opportunity to bring their insights to health care, but first they need to understand the industry and to speak its special language. Dr. Margaret Schulte has written the perfect book to bridge the gap. *Healthcare Delivery in the U.S.A.* is the resource that outsiders need to join the conversation and start teaching the medical sector lessons it must learn from other industries. The more non-health professionals who read this book, the sooner we'll see efficiency and effectiveness in medical care."

Jeff Bauer, Ph.D.
Management Consulting Partner and Director of the Futures Practice
Affiliated Computer Services Healthcare Solutions
Author of *Paradox and Imperatives in Health Care*

"I wish a book like this had been available when I entered health care. In easy-to-understand terms, Dr. Schulte lays out the components of the healthcare system so those of us who enter can be oriented to the terms and to the various entities we will be encountering. As the level of complexity of the healthcare system continues to increase, books such as this can help us deconstruct the system into understandable components. As we know, in order to improve, we must first understand. Dr. Schulte helps us understand."

Dean Bliss
LeanImprovement Specialist
Iowa Health System

"Selling technology solutions to hospitals is challenging because it requires knowing what's important to different people—patients, doctors, and employees—without any margin for error. Dr. Schulte's book is "Healthcare 101" for any sales professional striving to understand the healthcare industry. It couldn't be more timely with the new economic stimulus package which includes $20 billion for healthcare IT."

Linda Ewing
Regional Sales Director
Amcom Software

Healthcare Delivery in the U.S.A.

An Introduction

Margaret F. Schulte, DBA, FACHE

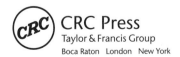

CRC Press
Taylor & Francis Group
Boca Raton London New York

CRC Press is an imprint of the
Taylor & Francis Group, an **informa** business
A PRODUCTIVITY PRESS BOOK

Productivity Press
Taylor & Francis Group
270 Madison Avenue
New York, NY 10016

© 2009 by Taylor and Francis Group, LLC
Productivity Press is an imprint of Taylor & Francis Group, an Informa business

---

Library of Congress Cataloging-in-Publication Data

Schulte, Maragaret F.
   Healthcare delivery in the U.S.A. : an introduction / Maragaret F. Schulte.
     p. ; cm.
   Includes bibliographical references and index.
   ISBN 978-1-4200-8493-1 (pbk. : alk. paper)
   1. Medical care--United States. I. Title. II. Title: Healthcare delivery in the USA.
   [DNLM: 1. Delivery of Health Care--United States. W 84 AA1 S386h 2010]

RA395.A3S38 2010
362.1--dc22
                                             2009028034

Visit the Taylor & Francis Web site at
http://www.taylorandfrancis.com

and the Productivity Press Web site at
http://www.productivitypress.com

Contents

Acknowledgments

The introduction refers to the fact that this book started years ago — in concept. There were so many people along the way who influenced my commitment to this work, and I would like to acknowledge and thank each one of them — the list would be too long — but that does not diminish their influence and inspiration. My friend and publisher, Kris Mednansky, is at the top of the list of the many to whom I owe gratitude — she has been patient with always a positive word; she has let me learn just what a book-writing adventure is all about. My graduate assistants, Uma Thandapeni and Hilary Jackson, have helped enormously: Uma in gathering an extensive amount of research, Hilary in expanding that research, creating tables and graphs, and keeping me organized. My students have provided constant inspiration, and my family has been a great influence — distracting me when I needed to get away from the book for a while but never begrudging the time it demanded of me. My many friends have shared my excitement and offered encouragement. Then there are my three little dogs (all rescue), Daney, Peaches, and Jimmy, who have lain by my feet for hours with endless patience — happy in their slumbers one moment and thrilled for the romps that cleared the webs from addled brains the next. Thank you, each and all.

Introduction

This book started some years ago, in work with students and so many others who have looked through the window into healthcare management, consulting, sales, and in other roles but have found a world that is complex and mystifying — one that in so many ways is confusing. As professionals have sought careers in healthcare whether with healthcare providers, payers, or vendors of technology, products and services, they too often "hit a wall" of isolation and confusion in which the lingo, structures, roles, relationships, and nuances of healthcare providers can be learned only through time spent "in the trenches" of experience. There are the professionals who work in one area of healthcare, whether clinical or administrative, and seek to stretch across the boundaries of their roles to new positions and opportunities. These persons also often face the complexities of what is effectively a new field of professional endeavor.

This book is for these individuals — it is meant to help them "jump start" their careers. Its mission is to provide the essentials for understanding and navigating the healthcare provider field. It is meant to provide the tools of understanding and knowledge. In it, the reader will walk through the history of the development of U.S. healthcare delivery and come to understand the highlights of a path that has shaped the strengths and weaknesses of a "system" that today is seen as too financially burdensome for the U.S. economy. The many venues of care delivery are described, and they provide a framework for understanding the fragmentation and lack of communication infrastructure that results in an environment ripe for errors and loss of the human connection that is the heart of care delivery.

Key to a successful and sustainable start in healthcare is an understanding of the wide array of people the professional will meet and work with in the provider organization. Clinicians and administrators come into healthcare from many different clinical, technical, management, and staff training programs and backgrounds. While we focus on the "major players" in the clinical setting (i.e., physicians, nurses, pharmacists and technologists), the role of clinicians and management becomes clear as the reader pages through the discussion of the structure of the system. This structure is different from so many other business enterprises — it is one in which physicians and hospitals, while integrally interdependent, also work at times at cross purposes — each holding to its own role and mission. It is here that the clinical and business sides of the healthcare enterprise occasionally clash and often find their stress points. It is also built on a third party payment system — one that drives a business model quite unlike that of other industries.

Healthcare, in the past decade, has come under a barrage of criticism following the 1999 release of the report *To Err is Human* of the Institutes of Medicine (IOM) — a report that confirmed that between 44,000 and 98,000 people die in hospitals each year due to preventable medical errors. Not only are people dying while in our care, many others are injured or are the fortunate ones who are the subject of "near misses" — in airline parlance, the accidents for which all the elements were right for catastrophe. The IOM report finally changed the fundamental way in which providers approach changes in their processes to weed out those preventable errors. It has driven a focus on information technology to gain more accurate and clear communication in the care setting. It has driven changes in reimbursement to deny payment to providers who must fix the results of preventable errors (e.g., when wrong site surgery is performed, the provider returns the patient to the operating room to perform right-site surgery). It has generated an expanded career field in healthcare — now populated with professionals dedicated to leading process change and to measuring results. It has led to public reporting of quality indicators, and publicly available comparisons of quality among competitive healthcare providers. Much more has changed with the issuance of the IOM report in 1999, and anyone coming into the field, whether with a vendor, provider, payer, or government organization, needs to understand the shifts that have occurred.

The financing of healthcare is a confusing mix of public and private programs. With the unabated rise in healthcare costs in the United States and the inauguration of a new President, a new focus on controlling costs is emerging. Old solutions are again being brought to the fore, and new solutions are being sought. This book does not address the possibilities of those solutions; its mission is to provide a basis for understanding the elements of the financing system today. We cannot be agents of change or effectively interact with healthcare providers and payers without an understanding of the basics of the current structures of payment.

Finally, we offer a glimpse into the research and medical science that is the pride of U.S. healthcare. The United States has been and continues to be a world leader in finding new cures and new technologies, in understanding the diseases and conditions to which our bodies are prone. There is promise here, and the opportunity that medicine presents to heal and cure the diseases we know of and those we have not yet discovered is awesome.

The individual's entry into healthcare will hopefully be made less turbulent and more successful with this book. It is meant to be a "quick read" one that paints a brief picture of healthcare in the United States today and provides a basis for interaction with providers from whatever perspective that interaction arises.

Now read on — I offer this as one tool for your success.

Chapter 1

History of the U.S. Healthcare Delivery System

1.1 Introduction

As we start the journey toward developing a better understanding of how healthcare delivery works in the United States, it is valuable to take a brief look backward and review the history that has shaped healthcare delivery. We see in today's healthcare the varied ideologies and philosophies, the evolving needs and wants, and the advances of generations past. We live with the decisions they made, and if we are to be involved in the evolution of the current system, then it behooves us to be aware of what shaped our current condition for better or for worse. For example, you may ask the question, "Why are employers in the United States so embedded in the financing of our healthcare through employee health insurance?" How did we get to the point at which employer-based health insurance has become such a negative burden on employers, for some of whom its costs are greater than the profit they earn? A quick look at history will show that during World War II, when federal mandates restricted employers from raising wages in light of looming rampant inflation, those employers turned to offering health insurance as a way of recruiting and retaining their workforce. It was a competitive move that, ironically, 75 years later, has created a competitive "stone around the neck" for those same employers as they try strategy after strategy to cut the costs of what once gave them competitive advantage. We need to understand a phenomenon such as this if we are to wisely and productively involve ourselves in healthcare today.

So, let us delve into that history. Healthcare delivery traces its roots back to the fourth century B.C., to Hippocrates, who is fondly referred to as the "father of medicine." However, we will not go back through the length of that rich past. Let us instead fast forward to a more recent time frame and start nearer the historic time in which our country was founded.

1.2   1750 to 1850 — The Early Days

In the early days of our country, there were no hospitals. People were reliant on itinerant physicians — some with legitimate, state-of-the-art-of-the-times medical education and others who took up the profession after serving as an apprentice. It was not until the latter half of the eighteenth century that our first hospitals developed. Contrary to the hospital we know today, those first hospitals were developed to house the "insane" and the poor when they came victim to life-threatening maladies or injuries. In growing cities, healthcare workers were able to work more efficiently when their patients were gathered in one place rather than spread throughout the city in homes and tenements. The Pennsylvania Hospital was built in Philadelphia in 1752, the New York Hospital was built in New Work City in 1771, and the Massachusetts Hospital was built in Boston in 1791 to improve worker productivity, advance medical delivery, and house those with mental or physical problems (1).

Among the major scientific advances of the times was the discovery of anesthesia in 1842. As we can only imagine, surgery before the availability of anesthesia was one of life's more horrendous events. Anesthesia not only brought relief to persons in dire need of surgery but also made it possible to have recourse to surgery earlier in the case of disease or injury — for example, before full limbs had to be removed due to infection.

A third major development in the delivery of medical care in the middle of the nineteenth century was the initiative of physicians to organize for the advancement of medicine and medical education. In 1847, the American Medical Association (AMA) was founded. With the founding of the AMA, a focus was brought to medical education and the improved training of doctors. An important implication of these early days of "professionalizing" medicine was the recognition of the need for structured and scientifically based medical education, for the sharing of medical knowledge, and for the documentation of the efficacy of new procedures.

1.3   1850 to the Late Nineteenth Century— Shift from Care to Cure

When we arrive at the Civil War period, some critical advances offered medicine the opportunity to again re-form its delivery. While previously hospitals had been primarily built and organized to house the terminally ill, the infectious, and the insane, the emphasis changed with the influx of the massive numbers of sick and injured soldiers and civilians. Medical advances of the time related to the discovery of bacteria and understanding the germ theory of disease. Anesthesia had just been discovered, and chloroform and ether became staples in surgical suites. Since an understanding of sepsis and infection was lacking, use of antiseptics was not to come until later. So the danger of the operating room still lurked — might the patient die of a disease other than that for which surgery was being performed (2)?

It would then stand to reason that the predominant health problems of the time related to infectious diseases. Although there were other kinds of health concerns, such as cardiovascular disease and cancer, deaths from infection were about twice as common as the "killer" diseases of today.

The Civil War provided, as wars always have, a "research laboratory" in which medical advances were achieved. On the battlefield, the demands of caring for the wounded became the necessity that is the "mother of invention." Civil War hospitals came to be seen as models of organization for medical delivery. Some of the contributions of the Civil War to medical delivery as we know it today include (1) the medical record in which data were systematically gathered, (2) the development of a system of managing mass casualties, (3) the pavilion-style general hospitals, which were well ventilated and clean, and copied in the design of large civilian hospitals over the next 75 years, (4) the importance of immediate, definitive treatment of wounds and fractures, (5) the importance of sanitation and hygiene in preventing infection, disease, and death, (6) the introduction of female nurses to hospital care, and (7) upgrading of the training of thousands of physicians and their introduction to new ideas and standards of care, such as prevention and treatment of infectious disease, anesthetic agents, and surgical standards that rapidly advanced the overall quality of American medical practice (3).

In 1860, bacteria were discovered as the source of disease. This laid the essential foundation for later discoveries in the control of infection. Advancements in understanding bacteria progressed quickly. With the use of that knowledge, the first bacteriological and chemical laboratory was organized in 1889; radiology followed in 1895.

Following the work of Florence Nightingale and other nursing pioneers, nurses were finally recognized and admitted to hospital care. However, their education was not yet organized within a formal educational curriculum. So, along with the recognition of nursing as a profession, a general call for improvements in nursing education and care was made, and the first school of nursing opened in 1872 at the New England Hospital for Women and Children. The establishment of additional schools of nursing followed shortly thereafter.

By the latter part of the nineteenth century, the role of hospitals began to change. They morphed from institutions focused on housing and care to become hospitals as we know them today — focused on cure. With the newly found understanding of infectious diseases and at least some limited ability to control them, hospitals were able to provide surgical procedures for more willing patients. Recognizing the need for ventilation and clean air, hospitals had some early and essential scientific tools to prevent illness. They no longer needed to simply serve as "warehouses" for the sick, and they were thus able to reshape their mission and role in society.

Physician training was far less organized then than it is today. In the mid–nineteenth century, there was no formal training program for physicians, so aspiring physicians were primarily educated by serving as apprentices. While those who could financially afford to do so went to major cities in Europe (e.g., Paris and London) to study and advance their medical education, others were more limited in what they could learn.

By the turn of the twentieth century, however, the training of physicians was recognized as a focal point for the improvement of medical care. A third major development in the delivery of medical care in the last half of the nineteenth century was the initiative of physicians to advance and improve medical education. New medical schools were developed. However, they were private, unsupervised, and lacked the structure needed for adequate medical training. As we will see later, these early steps in formalizing medical education were just that, *first steps* — steps that would face substantial reorganization in the early part of the next century.

1.4   1900 to the Mid–Twentieth Century— Era of Standardization

With the dawning of the twentieth century and the introduction of the "scientific method" in research, the pace of medical advances was accelerated. In 1907, Ross Harrison discovered how to grow living cells outside the body. His achievement opened the door to the study of living organisms at the cellular level. In 1912, cholesterol was found to be responsible for coronary artery disease, one of the major killers of the twentieth and twenty-first centuries. Sir Edward Banting led the team that discovered insulin in 1922, a discovery that had immediate impact globally for the masses of people who were wasting away with diabetes. Alexander Fleming, probably the best-known medical scientist of the era, discovered penicillin in 1928, a discovery that was to save thousands and thousands of lives during World War II after Pfizer perfected it for mass production.

Beyond medical discoveries, the early twentieth century found medical leaders taking up the cause of quality in medical delivery (an issue that the early twenty-first century finds us still trying to address). Hospitals were increasingly used by surgeons, and early on they took up the cause of improving outcomes of care. They turned first to the formalization of medical education. In 1910, the famed Flexner Report was released after 4 years of study under the leadership of Abraham Flexner. Among its findings were the quality of teaching in medical schools was poor, there was an absence of hospital-based training, and most medical graduates lacked adequate medical skills at graduation. Funded by the Carnegie Foundation, the Flexner Report called on American medical schools to adopt higher admission standards, stronger graduation standards, the grounding of medical training in the basic sciences, and for medical students to receive hospital-based training along with their classroom study. Many American medical schools fell short of the standard advocated in the report, and subsequent to its publication and at its recommendation, most medical schools in the United States were closed. The report also concluded that there were too many medical schools in the United States and that too many doctors were being trained — findings that also spurred the closing of medical schools (4).

Standardization impacted not only medical training but also the organization and operation of hospitals. Minimum standards of care in hospitals were published by the American College of Surgeons at approximately the same time as the Flexner Report was being completed. Shortly after the adoption of these minimum standards, a study to examine hospitals against the standards was undertaken, and it was found that of 692 hospitals examined, only 89 met all the standards. This ultimately led to the establishment of what is today The Joint Commission, a healthcare accrediting organization.

Standardization to improve outcomes of care impacted not only hospitals and physicians but also other clinical professionals. Professional licensing bodies grew during this time, and, ultimately, all professionals in clinical practice, physicians and others, were required to achieve professional licensure. The administration of licensure laws became the domain of individual states.

Mirroring the work of the AMA, the American Hospital Association was founded at the turn of the century as an organizational membership group through which public policy could be influenced and hospitals could share ideas and experiences.

Financially, healthcare delivery changed dramatically during the early twentieth century. With the founding of the prototype Blue Cross plan at Baylor University in Dallas, Texas, in 1929, the path was created for the rapid growth of health insurance and, decades later, for the sponsoring of health insurance as a benefit of employment.

While financing of medical care was spurred with new risk-sharing insurance plans and with the increased social acceptance of hospitals as places of cure and healing, advances in medical technology continued to impact the shaping of medical delivery. More sophisticated diagnostics and surgical procedures drove increased demand for facilities and technology, and the country needed to find a way to finance the construction of hospitals. The Hill-Burton Act, officially called the Hospital Survey and Construction Act, was passed in 1946 to fund the building of hospitals. Federal funds matched by local funding were provided to communities throughout the country to build and modernize hospitals. With a goal of having 4.5 hospital beds per 1000 population, there would be an expansion of almost 1000 hospitals over the next 25 years, as the number rose from 6125 in 1946 to 7123 in 1970 (Figure 1.1).

1.5 Mid-Twentieth Century to Present

Having come through the era of rapid growth in science and the ability to detect and treat disease and injury, the expansion of hospital facilities, the growth of health insurance, and the increased recognition of the need

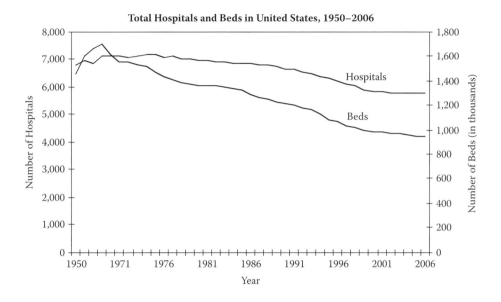

Figure 1.1 U.S. hospitals by number and bed size: 1950–2006. Source: Health Forum, American Hospital Association. "AHA Hospital Statistics." Health Forum LLC. 2008 Edition.

for government to play a larger role in assuring medical care for the poor, the late twentieth century was poised for further major change. While the healthcare sector grew, the demand for services also grew as the population played out its part in this expansionary sector of the economy. The post–World War II era saw the birth of the baby boom generation, and as lifestyles changed, the United States saw the emergence of a pattern of growth of chronic diseases, especially heart disease, stroke, and cancer. These major killers of the population continued their onward progress to afflict and consume a wide swath of the population over the next decades.

The latter half of the twentieth century was also a time of significant technological advances in medicine. In 1971, the computed tomographic scan was developed, and it was followed only 9 years later by the introduction of magnetic resonance imaging, which gave diagnosticians the ability to see the inside of the human body in ways that no other technology have previously provided. In the 1980s, the endoscope made it possible to enter the human body to perform diagnostics or surgical procedures with minimally invasive surgery.

In medical training, physicians sought out specialization. Medical schools and teaching hospitals expanded their programs to offer ever-increasing specialization training and make available some 145 specialties in which physicians can train, become certified, and enter professional practice. Likewise, clinical education for other professionals in healthcare grew expansively.

The combined interest in the expansion of the role of the American federal government in providing medical coverage for the poor and elderly came to its full fruition in the 1960s with the passage of Titles XVIII and XVIX (Medicare and Medicaid, respectively) of the Social Security Act. With the passage of Medicare (Title XVIII), individuals aged 65 years and older became entitled to the national health insurance program that Medicare continues to provide today; with the passage of Medicaid (Title XIX), the poor who met certain means-tested criteria (i.e., limited income and assets) gained access to medical care through a national health insurance program in which funding is shared by state and federal governments. In the decade after the introduction of Medicare, additional populations were brought under its coverage: persons with disabilities and persons with end-stage renal disease. Today, approximately 28% of the U.S. population is covered by these two national health insurance programs.

With the rapid expansion of commercial health insurance through employer-sponsored programs and the passage of Medicare and Medicaid, the costs of healthcare rose substantially. We cover this later in this book in a bit more detail. Suffice it to say at this point that the rise in the costs of healthcare delivery brought on a rash of legislative and regulatory attempts to curb the rate of increase. These attempts included the passage of cost containment acts to cut reimbursement levels and of certificate of need laws to control capital spending and expansion of services, passage of the prospective payment system, and expansion in the use of health maintenance organizations (HMOs) and of managed care concepts.

On another front, the last half of the twentieth century brought on another phenomenon — that of the growth of for-profit ownership and of multihospital companies. The United States, particularly in the south, had been accustomed to the presence of privately owned hospitals. In many small communities, the sole small hospital serving the community was owned by one or more doctors. However, with the passage of Medicare and Medicaid and their generous reimbursement of capital costs, the real estate and operational values of hospital properties were sufficient to entice investors to provide the capital and start-up costs for private, for-profit companies such as the Hospital Corporation of America, now The Hospital Company, and others to venture into hospital ownership on a large scale.

The rise of managed care in the last half of the twentieth century provided an alternative option for the control of rising healthcare costs. Under the Health Maintenance Organization Act of 1973, employers with 25 or more employees were required to offer their employees the option to join a federally certified HMO if such an HMO asked the employer to make its plan available to those employees. While HMOs offered more restrictive options in the choice of providers, they typically offered coverage with minimal out-of-pocket cost to the enrollee, which was be an attractive option to persons with constrained financial resources.

Advocates of health reform and market reform found early voice in the work of Alain Enthovan and his colleagues in the Jackson Hole Group. It was they who formalized the concept of "managed competition," which gradually morphed into "managed care." This was touted as the approach to healthcare delivery that would reduce the rise in healthcare costs and improve quality of care.

In discussing the rise of managed care, the rise of the integrated delivery system (IDS) or integrated delivery network (IDN) requires mention. The managed care environment found managed care companies approaching hospitals to negotiate rates at which they would pay for care for the people covered under their plans. With the concept that the managed care company would manage the care of the patient through case management the "other side of the coin" implied that costs would also be managed.

1.6   Competition

Competition between providers and payers intensified during the 1990s, as each vied for the private paying patient and for the more lucrative diagnostic and surgical procedures, such as orthopedics and cardiac care. In a public policy environment that favored competition as a way to reduce costs, hospitals expanded their sophisticated services, such as CT scanning and open heart surgery, and developed specialized services to gain deeper market penetration. Physicians sought new areas of specialization as technology advanced, and that specialization sparked even more competition as hospitals sought to gain competitive advantage. In this environment, marketing became a buzzword and soon a new science in the management of hospitals.

Managed care lent its own brand of competitiveness to healthcare providers. As managed care organizations grew to represent increasing numbers of "covered lives," their ability to gain deep discounts from providers that would join their "network" also grew. In a corresponding effort to gain strength at the negotiating table, major hospitals moved to create IDNs or IDSs by acquiring, developing, or merging with other hospitals, nursing facilities, ambulatory care centers, rehabilitation centers, specialty hospitals, diagnostic centers, freestanding laboratories and radiology centers, and physician practices. These IDNs not only offered greater strength at the negotiating table when managed care companies were on the other side of the table but also offered the opportunity to capture markets on the premise that they could offer the full "continuum of services" that a patient might need. Patients could be referred within the healthcare system for whatever they needed — theoretically simplifying each patient's life (although, lacking true organizational integration, this did not materialize) and ensuring that the patient would stay within the system.

Public and private investments in medical research resulted in dramatic advances in pharmaceuticals during the decades of the late 1900s. The Human Genome Project, and private researchers finally broke the code of DNA, our genetic makeup, creating the path to a whole field of new and potential breakthroughs in medicine.

1.7   Summary

From the time of the early founding of the United States, healthcare grew and changed as dramatically as other sectors of society. Despite setbacks along the way, the advances in science moved from an understanding of sepsis and its relationship to infection and death to an ability to perform multiple-organ transplant and to understanding the genome, hospital organizations changed from the poor houses of the eighteenth century to the highly sophisticated organizations that they are today. Physician training went from the haphazard arena of apprenticeship to the disciplined and lengthy course of education of today's medical schools; payment structure went from the bartering model of the early days of the country to today's multitrillion dollar third-party payment system; the legal dimension of healthcare grew and became more complex and demanding, and government involvement intensified. We discuss each of these as we continue through the next chapters.

References

1. J. B. Cutter, 1933. "Early hospital history in the United States." *California Journal of Medicine*, 20(8): 272–274. Available at: http://www.pubmedcentral.nih.gov/pagerender.fcgi?artid=1517304&pageindex=2
2. University of Victoria, Canada, 2008. "Medicine in 1860s Victoria: 19th century medicine." Accessed September 2008. Available at: http://web.uvic.ca/vv/student/medicine/medicine19c.htm
3. F. W. Blaisdell, 1988. "Medical advances during the Civil War." *Archives of Surgery*, 123(9): 1045–1050.
4. H. Beck, 2004. "The Flexner Report and the standardization of American medical education." *Journal of American Medical Association*, 291:2139–2140. Accessed September 2008. Available at: http://jama.ama-assn.org/cgi/content/full/291/17/2139

Websites

Centers for Disease Control and Prevention (CDC): http://www.cdc.gov
World Health Organization (WHO): http://www.who.int

Chapter 2

Health Status
The Health of the Population

2.1 Introduction

The World Health Organization, in its constitution, defines health as the "the state of complete physical, mental, and social well-being" (1). Today, that definition continues to be used as the all-encompassing definition of health. It describes the ideal state or condition of each human being. However, achieving that ideal state is subject to interpretation and challenge. As this definition is applied, whether individually or by society, the application occurs within limitations — the limitations of scarce resources that would be needed to fully accomplish such a state of health, of incomplete knowledge, and of lack of public will to sacrifice and change priorities to fully achieve the World Health Organization's definition of the individual human condition. In the public policy realm, "health" is inherently defined narrowly by the limitation of resources to allocate to health and by the balancing of social and national priorities. Implicitly, then, society accepts a definition of health that is within the financial capacity and will of that society to provide for the health needs of its populations. It is also defined narrowly by individuals who are influenced by their economic, educational, and social status and by their views. Those who are wealthy and well educated, for example, tend to enjoy better health and better access to medical care.

There is also the question of what "health" means to individuals. What is defined as complete well-being for the individual with a genetic propensity toward a particular disease may be different from the individual who has been permanently injured in an accident or who has been the subject of physical or emotional violence. The term "health" takes on different interpretations based on our individual and communal perspectives.

■ From an individual perspective, our interest is in maintaining our health and in keeping ourselves free of injury and illness, and when we suffer the misfortune of injury or disease, we want to know that there is medical care available and accessible to overcome that misfortune. However, disparities in access to medical care exist in our society, and we do not all share equally in the "promise of healthcare." There are many who do not have the financial or geographic access to health services that many of us enjoy.

■ From a community perspective, we look to environmental and population-based approaches to achieve health goals. In our various communities, we typically are groups of people with something in common, whether that be geography, race, employment, religious belief, or some other bonding characteristic. It is these shared communities that shape our medical delivery. Healthcare is a local service, and as such it is shaped by the resources and demands of local wants and needs.

2.2 Health Status

"Health status" is one of the key measures of the "health" of a society. Health status is measured from a variety of factors; however, the primary measures used are mortality (death) rates, morbidity (illness) rates, life expectancy, and infant mortality rates. As Jonas and Kovner (2) said, "there are not as yet any generally accepted direct measures of health" (p. 16), so we continue to rely on the traditional measures of mortality and morbidity.

2.3 Mortality

1. Mortality rates are the measure of deaths within a population overall and from particular causes.
   – As would be expected, these rates have changed over the years as medical care has improved. Generally, we are living longer, and we die less frequently from the infectious diseases of the past. Instead, we face death more frequently from other conditions such as heart disease, diabetes, and cancer. According to the National Center for Health Statistics, the overall mortality rate in the United States has trended downward since 1980, as shown in Table 2.1. A more

detailed look at the data in Table 2.2, provided by the Centers for Disease Control (CDC), reflects disparities in mortality rates between races by geography. Residents of the East South Central U.S. tend to have higher mortality rates, particularly among Black or African-Americans than any other region or race in the country. We address these disparities a bit later in this chapter.

Table 2.1 Mortality Rates for US Population
per 100,000 population

Year	Overall	Male	Female
1980	1039.1	1348.1	817.9
1990	938.7	1202.8	750.9
2000	869.0	1053.8	731.4
2004	800.8	955.7	679.2

Source: Kung HC, Hoyert DL, Xu JQ, Murphy SL. Deaths: Final data for 2005. National vital statistics reports; vol 56 no 10. Hyattsville, MD: National Center for Health Statistics. 2008.

Table 2.2 Mortality Rates for the US Population by Race and Geography
per 100,000 population

Geographic Division and State	All Persons	White	Black or African American	American Indian or Alaska Native	Asian or Pacific Islander	Hispanic or Latino	White, not Hispanic or Latino
United States	826.5	811.0	1,059.7	671.2	460.9	613.9	820.3
New England	767.9	769.4	843.2	*	364.2	516.7	768.5
Middle Atlantic	793.7	787.2	918.0	*	380.5	565.5	790.0
East North Central	848.7	824.2	1,114.6	*	373.5	521.9	826.9
West North Central	797.9	783.8	1,096.4	*	433.6	561.4	780.7
South Atlantic	844.5	806.1	1,073.1	*	367.5	573.4	820.3
East South Central	981.8	951.3	1,163.9	*	406.6	380.7	954.3
West South Central	894.9	870.6	1,151.7	*	418.2	691.5	897.9
Mountain	796.9	794.2	956.4	867.9	472.3	731.6	795.2
Pacific	748.4	765.8	1,007.3	*	511.6	592.9	788.4

Source: National Center for Health Statistics. Health United States, 2007: With Chartbook on Trends in the Health of Americans. Table 28. Hyattsville, MD: 2006.

– Within mortality statistics are the data that tell us the major reasons for those deaths. While the proportions of deaths caused by diseases of the heart and those caused by cerebrovascular disease have decreased in the last half century, they are still the dominant causes of death. Of note, U.S. death rates from cancer (malignant neoplasms) have not changed much over the last 50 years. The CDC reports the rates per 100,000 population (Table 2.3). The CDC's National Center for Vital Statistics reports the causes of death in terms of deaths as a percentage of total deaths in the United States. The top ten leading causes of death are reported in Table 2.4.

2. Life expectancy rates are directly related to mortality. Life expectancy statistics reflect the average life span of individuals from selected starting points, such as birth or age 65 years. In other words, if one lives to age 65 years, then the average life expectancy data will tell that person what life span he or she might have from that point forward, all things being equal (Figure 2.1). This is an average only, and each individual's life span may vary depending on factors such as health status at age 65 years and subsequent injury or disease. As mortality statistics have decreased overall, life expectancy statistics shown significant improvement over the past decades. In other words, people in the United States are living longer today

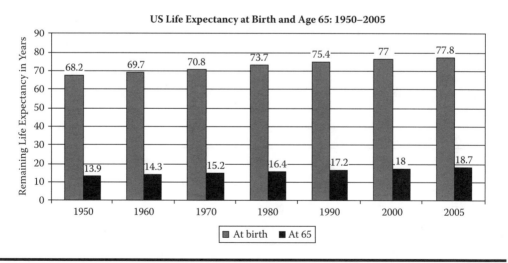

Figure 2.1   U.S. life expectancy at birth and age 65 years: 1950–2005. Source: National Center for Health Statistics. *Health United States, 2007: With Chartbook on Trends in the Health of Americans.* Hyattsville, MD: National Center for Health Statistics, 2007.

Table 2.3 Causes of Death in the United States
per 100,00 population

Cause of Death	1950	2000	2005
Heart Disease	586.8	257.6	211.1
Cerebrovascular Disease	180.7	60.9	46.6
Malignant Neoplasms	193.9	199.6	183.8

Source: Kung HC, Hoyert DL, Xu JQ, Murphy SL. Deaths: Final data for 2005. National vital statistics reports; Vol. 56, No. 10. Hyattsville, MD: National Center for Health Statistics. 2008.

Table 2.4 U.S. Leading Causes of Death: 2005

Cause of Death	Total Deaths	Percent of Total
All causes	2,448,017	100.0
Diseases of heart	652,091	26.6
Malignant neoplasms (cancers)	559,312	22.8
Cerebrovascular diseases	143,579	5.9
Chronic lower respiratory diseases	130,933	5.3
Accidents (unintentional injuries)	117,809	4.8
Diabetes mellitus	75,119	3.1
Alzheimer's disease	71,599	2.9
Influenza and pneumonia	63,001	2.6
Nephritis, nephrotic syndrome and nephrosis	43,901	1.8
Septicemia	34,136	1.4
Intentional self-harm (suicide)	32,637	1.3
Chronic liver disease and cirrhosis	27,530	1.1
Essential (primary hypertension and hypertensive renal disease	24,902	1.0
Parkinson's disease	19,544	0.8
Assault (homicide)	18,124	0.7
All other cause (residual)	433,800	17.7

Source: Kung HC, Hoyert DL, Xu JQ, Murphy SL. Deaths: Final data for 2005. National vital statistics reports; Vol. 56, No. 10. Hyattsville, MD: National Center for Health Statistics. 2008.

than they did a decade or more ago. The CDC reports that life expectancy at birth in 1900 was 47.3 years, but by 2004, this statistical average had increased to 77.8 years (3). Overall, life expectancy rates at birth and by gender are shown in Table 2.5. In a continuing pattern, women tend to live longer than men. The 2005 data indicate a >5 year longer life span, on average, for women.

3. Infant mortality rate is another important measure of our health status. It is defined as "the number of deaths under the age of one year among children born alive, divided by the number of live births" (2). The United States has a higher overall infant mortality rate than might be expected. As Jonas and Kovner (2) explained, there is a major discrepancy in infant mortality rates in the United States among population groups based on ethnicity, education, and wealth. The National Center for Health Statistics reported that the overall infant mortality rate for the United States was 6.9 per 1000 live births in 2000. When these data are analyzed relative to infant mortality among blacks and whites in the United States, the statistics are significantly different. In 2000, there were 14.0 infant deaths per 1000 live births among the black population as compared with 5.7 among the white population.

With its high infant mortality rate, the United States takes a "back seat" to many other developed countries in the world. In 2004, the United States ranked forty-second in world infant mortality, behind Cuba and Taiwan and a host of other countries (National Center for Vital Health Statistics, 2007). Not only does the United States rank twenty-ninth among developed countries, but this ranking has fallen over the past several decades. In 1960, the United States' international ranking was twelfth, but it fell to twenty-third in 1990 and to twenty-ninth in 2004 (Table 2.6).

Table 2.5 Life Expectancy at Birth for U.S. Population

Year	Overall	Male	Female
1900	47.3	46.3	48.3
1950	68.2	65.6	71.1
2000	77.0	74.3	79.7
2004	77.8	75.2	80.4

Source: National Center for Health Statistics. *Health United States, 2007: With Chartbook on Trends in the Health of Americans.* Hyattsville, MD: National Center for Health Statistics, 2007.

Table 2.6 Comparative Infant Mortality Statistics: 2008

Rank	Country	Infant Mortality Rate (deaths per 1,000 live births)	Rank	Country	Infant Mortality Rate deaths per 1,000 live births
1	Singapore	2.3	26	Netherlands	4.81
2	Sweden	2.75	27	Australia	4.82
3	Japan	2.8	28	Portugal	4.85
4	Hong Kong	2.93	29	Gibraltar	4.91
5	Macau	3.23	30	United Kingdom	4.93
6	Iceland	3.25	31	New Zealand	4.99
7	France	3.36	32	Jersey	5.01
8	Finland	3.5	33	Canada	5.08
9	Anguilla	3.54	34	Ireland	5.14
10	Norway	3.61	35	Monaco	5.18
11	Andorra	3.68	36	Greece	5.25
12	Malta	3.79	37	San Marino	5.44
13	Czech Republic	3.83	38	Taiwan	5.45
14	Germany	4.03	39	Italy	5.61
15	Switzerland	4.23	40	Isle of Man	5.62
16	Spain	4.26	41	Cuba	5.93
17	Israel	4.28	42	United States	6.3
18	Korea, South	4.29	43	European Union	6.38
19	Slovenia	4.3	44	Faroe Islands	6.46
20	Denmark	4.4	45	Croatia	6.49
21	Austria	4.48	46	Belarus	6.53
22	Belgium	4.5	47	Guam	6.55
23	Liechtenstein	4.52	48	Lithuania	6.57
24	Guernsey	4.53	49	Northern Mariana Islands	6.72
25	Luxembourg	4.62	50	Cyprus	6.75

Source: Central Intelligence Agency, United States. "World Factbook, Rank Order—Infant Mortality Rate." 2008 est. Accessed January 2009. https://www.cia.gov/library/publications/the-world-factbook/rankorder/2091rank.html

2.4 Morbidity

Morbidity statistics identify the major illnesses from which we suffer as a population. Morbidity statistics are reported both in terms of prevalence of a disease (total number of cases in a specific time frame) and in terms of the incidence of a disease (number of new cases of a disease in a specific time frame). As we begin to look at morbidity data, we see the level of chronic diseases that characterize our population. These include such conditions as diabetes, obesity, and back pain, among others. Figure 2.2 provides the U.S. morbidity statistics relative to the prevalence of disabilities and associated health conditions.

The difficulty in getting accurate data results from the problem of gaining accurate reporting of morbidity data across the range of possible conditions to which any population is subject. For example, reporting is inconsistent due to patients not seeking care, their reticence to report diseases for fear of reprisal, such as loss of a job, and the fact that the only data in national reports are those from MDs and DOs. Additionally, with the widespread use of alternative therapies (such as homeopathy), there are morbidity data that never get reported.

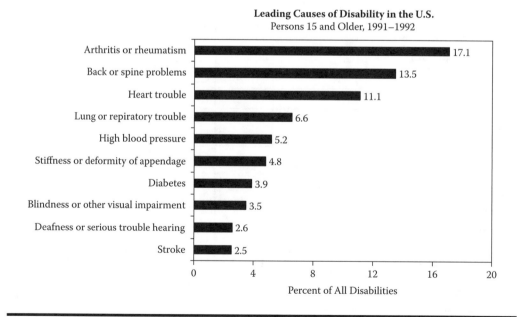

Leading Causes of Disability in the U.S.
Persons 15 and Older, 1991–1992

Figure 2.2 **Leading cause of disability in the United States. Source: Centers for Disease Control and Prevention. Prevalence of disabilities and associated health conditions — United States, 1991–1992.** *Morbidity and Mortality Weekly Reports.* **43(40):730–731, 737–739, 1994.**

2.5 Health Determinants

Health determinants are those factors that affect our individual health status and that of populations. For example, if a group of individuals resides in an environmentally unsafe geographic area, it is likely that the health of those individuals will be at risk and that the health of a number of them will be negatively impacted by that environment. Health determinants are composed of biological, environmental, medical, and social factors. Table 2.8 identifies the categories of these factors and the subfactors that make up each category.

"The Lalonde report of 1974 (issued by then Canadian Minister of National Health and Welfare, Marc Lalonde) popularized the idea that direct medical care might be but a bit player in producing and reducing mortality. That report highlighted the fact that other factors — biology, environment, lifestyle — figure more prominently than medical care in producing health" (4).

Biological factors are those with which we are born. They are composed of heredity and genetics, both of which impact our propensity to succumb to certain diseases. They also affect our physical characteristics, such as whether we are tall or short, blonde or dark haired, and so on. Advances in the science of genetics offer the potential to reshape some of those characteristics through, for example, embryonic gene transplantation.

Environmental factors are those of our physical environment, the sociocultural impact of our primary and other reference groups, economic conditions that impact us directly, and education. Studies have shown repeatedly that education and income are directly related to a more positive health status in a given population.

The availability and scope of medical services available to us also influence our health status. While we in the United States are privileged to have incredibly advanced medical science available, we know that all of those advancements are not available to all of our citizens. Those who do not have access, whether due to geography or indigence, tend to have poorer overall health status than those who have access to care.

Table 2.8 Health Determinants

• Biological
– Heredity
– Genetics
• Environmental
– Physical
– Sociocultural
– Economic
– Education
• Medical
– Health services utilized
• Social
– Lifestyle
– Behavior

Social factors are those related to lifestyle and behavior. They include, for instance, how and what we eat (e.g., a diet of fast foods or high-carbohydrate and/or high-fat foods is linked to obesity and heart disease), our compliance with safety laws (e.g., wearing seatbelts), getting sufficient sleep, minimizing stress, performing in dangerous occupations, lack of exercise, and smoking.

Among the social factors that influence health status are the sociodemographics of the population. These include:

■ Population growth: As the population grows, demand for goods and services increases and the need for jobs expands; if productivity or availability of goods and services does not keep pace with population growth, prices rise and income falls.

■ Aging baby boomers: It is expected that the aging baby boom population will require more healthcare services as their health conditions deteriorate. While this population generally will be healthier longer, in their later years, the need for primary health services, particularly, will expand. The United States is not keeping pace with the supply of primary care practitioners, and will face a significant shortage if solutions are not implemented now to incentivize medical students to focus on primary care.

■ Growth in ethnic populations: As ethnic populations grow in the United States, so will the demand for services to meet their unique needs. For example, hospitals and other healthcare providers serving ethnic populations need multilingual staff.

■ Population mobility: Population mobility, particularly as people move for jobs or to spend time in warmer weather regions, impacts the need for seasonal capacity expansion in those areas. When capacity depends primarily on a trained workforce, the ability to meet those capacity requirements is challenged in areas that experience seasonal contraction and expansion of the population.

■ Income gap widening between richest and poorest.

■ Persistent poverty: As poverty and joblessness have increased, so have the ranks of the uninsured. On the one hand, those without health insurance tend to put off treatment until they find themselves in an emergency room, which is far more costly than the primary care that might have prevented a serious medical problem. On the other hand, those without health insurance tend to seek out emergency rooms to provide basic care, knowing that the emergency room cannot, under law, turn them away. This is an expensive source of basic healthcare service.

2.6   Summary

Health status refers to the condition of the health of a population. An understanding of health status is central to the design of a system that can address the major health issues of a given population. Comparative health statistics in particular paint a picture of those areas in which gains have been achieved and in which the country may need to reprioritize the use of resources. Over the past century, the life span of the U.S. population has increased significantly. However, there is still a disparity between the shorter average life span of men compared to that of women. Infant mortality rates position the United States far below other countries in the world — infants younger than 1 year have a higher probability of dying than do infants in 42 other countries. When the U.S. population is analyzed by specific subgroups, the data indicate that those of nonwhite ethnic populations tend to have a much higher infant mortality rate than the white population. It is these disparities toward which public health programs are targeted and for which research has been under way to better understand and to design programs that can reverse the causes of the disparities.

References

1. World Health Organization, 2006. "Constitution of the World Health Organization." Accessed January 2009. Available at: http://www.who.int/ governance/eb/who_constitution_en.pdf
2. A. R. Kovner and J. R. Knickman (Editors), 2008. *Jonas & Kovner's Health Care Delivery in the United States*, 9th Edition. Springer: New York.
3. National Center for Health Statistics, 2007. "Health United States, 2006: With Chartbook on Trends in the Health of Americans." National Center for Health Statistics: Hyattsville, MD. Available at: http://www.cdc.gov/nchs/data/hus/ hus06.pdf#027
4. Project Hope, 2008. "Prologue: The social determinants of health." *Health Affairs*, 27(2): 320.

Websites

Centers for Disease Control and Prevention (CDC): http://www.cdc.gov
National Center for Vital Health Statistics: http://www.cdc/gov/nchs
World Health Organization (WHO): http://www.who.int

Chapter 3

Components of the Healthcare Delivery System

3.1 Introduction

The structure of healthcare delivery is composed of an array of organizations and professionals, each of whom brings value to the ultimate outcome of medical care. Healthcare is a "local business," and as such, this sector of our society and economy is impacted by the fragmentation of a wide array of unconnected providers and payers. This fragmentation brings a number of challenges to healthcare delivery and outcomes. We address these in this chapter, but, first, let us reach an understanding of the central players who provide medical care.

When we think of healthcare providers, hospitals and doctors come to mind. However, there are many other providers of healthcare (long-term nursing homes, home healthcare, diagnostic services, rehabilitation, ambulatory care, mini-clinics, mental health and substance abuse programs, etc.). Over the past decades of the expansion of managed care, healthcare providers have, on a local or regional level, aggregated into various types of "integrated delivery networks" in order to position themselves for more balanced managed care contracting, to retain and expand market share and, for some, to grow in size to support and own managed care functions.

We first discuss the types of providers and provider organizations that are available and then look at the integration of those providers in chapter 4.

3.2 Who Are the Players in Healthcare Delivery?

3.2.1 Healthcare Providers: Inpatient or Outpatient?

Healthcare providers are often classified according to the type of care they provide or, considered from another perspective, by the condition of the patients they serve. Providers classified to be of "acute care" are those who provide "medical services for persons with or at risk for acute or active medical conditions in a variety of ambulatory and inpatient settings" (1). In other words, acute care encompasses services that meet serious episodic needs, such as those arising from injuries and diseases that are subject to cure through surgical, pharmaceutical, or other therapeutic approaches.

Acute care is provided, as Jonas and Kovner suggest, in the inpatient or ambulatory setting. Distinction between these two settings might best be described in terms of the patient: in the inpatient setting, the patient stays overnight; in the ambulatory, or outpatient, setting, the patient does not stay overnight — he or she walks (or ambulates) in and out of the medical care venue on the same day. Inpatients undergo more intensive round-the-clock medical care until their discharge from the hospital.

Due to the scientific and procedural advances of the past several decades (discussed in chapter 1), many procedures that once required inpatient admission to a hospital are now performed in the ambulatory arena. Laser surgery and endoscopy, for example, have allowed physicians to perform minimally invasive procedures with local anesthetics. The patient is able to recover comfortably and safely at home after undergoing surgery in which the physician used very small incisions. Thus, increasing numbers of surgical procedures have moved from the inpatient to the outpatient, or ambulatory, setting.

3.2.2 Scope and Size of Hospitals

Hospitals range in size from the very small to the major academic medical centers and government-owned facilities that may primarily serve indigents or other population groups. In all, there were 5,747 hospitals in the United States in 2006. These are operated as community hospitals, federal government hospitals, nonfederal psychiatric hospitals, nonfederal long-term care hospitals and units of institutions, such as prisons and college infirmaries (Table 3.1).

Hospitals are typically categorized by the number of beds they are licensed to operate and, in a secondary measure, by the number of beds they

Table 3.1 Number of U.S. Hospitals: 2006

Total Number of All U.S. Registered* Hospitals	5747
Number of U.S. Community** Hospitals	4 927
Number of Nongovernment Not-for-Profit Community Hospitals	2919
Number of Investor-Owned (For-Profit) Community Hospitals	889
Number of State and Local Government Community Hospitals	1119
Number of Rural Community Hospitals	2001
Number of Urban Community Hospitals	2926
Number of Federal Government Hospitals	221
Number of Nonfederal Psychiatric Hospitals	451
Number of Nonfederal Long-Term Care Hospitals	129
Number of Hospital Units of Institutions (Prison Hospitals, College Infirmaries, etc.)	19

*Hospitals that meet American Hospital Association criteria for registration as a
     hospital facility.
**All nonfederal, short-term general, and other special hospitals.
Sourec: American Hospital Association. "Fast Facts on U.S. Hospitals." Updated
     October 2007. http://www.aha.org/aha/resource-center/Statistics-and-Studies/
     fast-facts.html

have in operation, termed "staffed beds." The distinction between licensed and staffed beds relates to the fact that a hospital may not have all of its licensed beds in use at any point in time. When a hospital experiences an inpatient utilization level that is substantially below the licensed number of beds it operates, it will tend to take some of the beds out of service. This allows for improved operational and cost efficiency, and it allows the hospital to retain the right, under its license, to reopen beds if and when they are needed. Figure 3.1 reflects the reduction in both numbers of hospitals since their high number of over 7000 in the 1970s to less than 6000 in 2006. It also offers a view of the number of beds in operation in the United States and the sharp reduction in beds that has occurred since the highs of the 1960s. At that time, the U.S. had approximately 1700 acute care beds per 1000 population. This ratio dropped to a low of about 900 per 1000 population.

Table 3.2 offers a listing of the number of hospitals in each state, U.S. territory, and the District of Columbia, the number of staffed beds, discharges, utilization by patient days, and gross patient revenue for 2006. From this chart, the reader can easily calculate the average length of stay (ALOS) in each state by dividing patient days by total discharges. ALOS is an important statistic to hospital management because reimbursement by Medicare

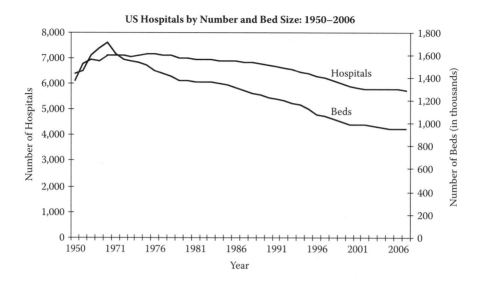

Figure 3.1 U.S. hospitals by number and bed size: 1950–2006. Source: Health Forum, American Hospital Association. "AHA Hospital Statistics." Health Forum LLC. 2008 Edition.

Table 3.2 List of U.S. Hospitals by Number, Utilization and Gross Patient Revenue, 2006

State	Number of Hospitals	Staffed Beds	Total Discharges	Patient Days	Gross Patient Revenue
Alaska	16	1,098	36,819	239,955	$2,037,329
Alabama	101	15,942	639,569	3,551,887	$27,353,632
Arkansas	54	7,901	321,985	1,676,865	$11,561,411
Arizona	71	11,537	667,898	2,922,675	$29,983,571
California	365	75,605	3,221,821	18,549,541	$204,359,794
Colorado	54	8,284	400,355	1,961,465	$21,600,714
Connecticut	34	8,388	385,990	2,405,235	$17,382,656
Washington DC	9	2,748	121,201	814,480	$6,120,478
Delaware	8	2,170	98,644	583,380	$3,106,345
Florida	211	52,586	2,356,252	12,295,786	$119,249,102
Georgia	116	23,241	901,456	5,977,878	$38,756,159
Guam	2	179	11,262	57,362	$120,673
Hawaii	15	2,718	92,137	756,339	$4,145,032
Iowa	39	7,375	278,733	1,606,078	$11,123,831
Idaho	19	2,272	111,003	486,902	$3,541,020
Illinois	144	32,341	1,440,409	7,789,574	$69,615,759
Indiana	89	16,697	663,786	3,597,968	$28,793,800
Kansas	59	6,652	286,979	1,407,627	$12,634,388

Table 3.2 *continued*

Kentucky	76	13,146	556,565	3,091,886	$21,977,496
Louisiana	113	15,481	583,739	3,279,728	$23,054,469
Massachusetts	82	15,064	755,559	4,087,048	$34,947,980
Maryland	51	11,661	734,023	3,356,419	$13,521,012
Maine	23	3,140	127,439	736,719	$5,153,699
Michigan	115	23,476	1,080,729	5,872,599	$48,402,494
Minnesota	55	10,632	516,989	2,709,071	$20,455,988
Missouri	91	17,835	714,989	3,972,637	$33,201,899
Mississippi	73	11,159	379,544	2,277,998	$15,020,353
Montana	20	2,440	81,158	589,531	$3,013,669
North Carolina	109	22,866	986,478	5,966,090	$38,077,440
North Dakota	17	2,297	73,395	543,256	$2,793,350
Nebraska	24	4,463	170,300	1,091,279	$7,750,373
New Hampshire	14	2,199	99,683	534,062	$5,347,015
New Jersey	75	21,230	1,041,893	5,838,001	$68,182,932
New Mexico	39	3,846	161,924	808,361	$6,991,805
Nevada	29	4,858	272,174	1,318,003	$14,481,524
New York	214	61,956	2,203,633	18,260,835	$101,505,387
Ohio	150	30,563	1,372,355	7,279,353	$63,488,311
Oklahoma	100	10,634	449,377	2,363,826	$17,092,498
Oregon	35	5,819	304,904	1,439,313	$11,939,236
Pennsylvania	182	37,007	1,675,236	9,601,106	$102,856,438
Puerto Rico	53	8,003	387,112	2,239,123	$3,654,511
Rhode Island	12	2,510	131,326	703,068	$6,085,979
South Carolina	63	11,742	512,441	3,004,575	$23,733,528
South Dakota	29	2,662	83,808	653,801	$3,253,712
Tennessee	122	20,246	816,379	4,609,973	$34,585,608
Texas	366	55,666	2,524,963	12,521,117	$116,432,083
Utah	35	3,968	195,910	933,693	$6,579,379
Virginia	91	19,320	744,312	4,758,509	$32,753,094
Vermont	7	825	37,418	205,218	$2,121,714
Washington	61	9,329	515,325	2,334,663	$24,615,410
Wisconsin	73	11,343	525,378	2,537,532	$22,310,259
West Virginia	41	6,434	245,569	1,473,969	$8,057,121
Wyoming	15	1,224	39,600	249,031	$1,296,752
Totals	4,061	762,778	33,137,926	187,922,390	$1,556,220,213

Source: American Hospital Directory. "Hospital Statistics by State." Web-accessed, 2008. http://www.ahd.com/state_statistics.html

and other payers is designed to disincentivize costly, unnecessary days of hospitalization.

ALOS is a basic statistic that hospitals monitor on an ongoing basis. This information indicates how long, on average, patients are staying in a hospital as inpatients. This information is reviewed not only for the over-all hospital but also for the various inpatient services within the hospital, such as intensive care units, neonatal intensive care units, orthopedics and pediatrics. Figure 3.2 indicates that the overall ALOS for U.S. hospitals in 2006 was 5.6 days. As noted in the figure, the ALOS for U.S. hospitals has been decreasing steadily since 1983, when it was 7.6 days. This decrease is due to the increased use of ambulatory and outpatient procedures and to reductions in reimbursement for many inpatient stays.

Gross patient revenues are also included in Figure 3.2. It should be noted that the dollars stated in the table do not include revenue from other sources. These may include earnings on investments, rental income, bequests, and donations, and income from other nonpatient operations, such as parking lots and food services to visitors and staff.

3.2.3 Levels of Care

Medical care is provided at different levels of sophistication, depending on the severity and complexity (i.e., acuity) of a patient's injury or illness. These

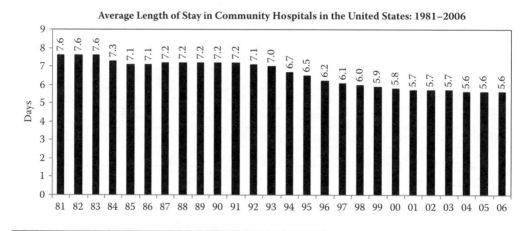

Figure 3.2 Average length of stay in community hospitals in the United States: 1981–2006. American Hospital Association: http://www.aha.org/aha/research-and-trends/chartbook/ch3.html. Source: Avalere Health Analysis of American Hospital Association Annual Survey data, 2006, for community hospitals (AHA web site).

levels of care are identified by the categories of primary, secondary, tertiary, and quaternary care. While major hospitals and teaching or academic health centers may offer all four levels of care, other hospitals may provide care up to the secondary or tertiary level and, in some rural areas where resources are lacking, others may limit their services to primary care.

The most basic services fall under the categorization of primary care. At this level, uncomplicated broken bones are set, minimal "simple" surgical procedures are done, general diagnostic work is provided, treatment of common ailments is offered, uncomplicated maternal and child services are provided, and other basic services are performed. Hospitals providing primary care may offer basic surgical services, such as appendectomies and setting of compound fractures, and other inpatient services for persons with chronic problems, the elderly, and others who may need observation and treatment in an inpatient setting. In addition to an outpatient department (OPD), many primary care hospitals also have an emergency department (ED) in which patients can be either stabilized and referred to a secondary- or tertiary-level hospital, or treated, if the presenting problem is uncomplicated. Roemer's model of health services systems defines primary care as the entry point into the health services system, wherein:

- illness or disease is diagnosed and initial treatment provided;
- episodic care for common, non-chronic illnesses and injuries is rendered;
- prescription drugs to treat common illnesses or injuries are provided;
- routine dental care occurs; and
- potentially serious physical or mental health conditions that require prompt referral for secondary or tertiary care are diagnosed (2).

The U.S. Institute of Medicine defines primary care as "the provision of integrated, accessible healthcare services by clinicians who are accountable for addressing a large majority of personal healthcare needs, developing a sustained partnership with patients, and practicing in the context of family and community" (3).

Primary care is also a designation used for physicians in specialties related to the services listed above. Primary care physicians include those in general internal medicine, family practice, general obstetrics and gynecology, and general pediatrics. While physicians in these specialties may also function at a secondary level of care (e.g., the pediatrician who diagnoses and treats a child with a more complicated medical problem), the dominant volume of their work is in primary care.

Primary care is offered in a variety of venues from the acute care setting to the well-baby clinic. Primary care hospitals provide basic inpatient services. Outpatient centers, ambulatory care, physician offices, community health organizations, diagnostic centers, surgery centers, home health services and long-term care facilities are all sites in which primary care is provided. While a number of these venues of care, such as outpatient centers, provide primary care, they may also provide some secondary care services, such as invasive specialty surgical procedures. In other words, some healthcare facilities are not exclusively dedicated to primary care; they may also offer secondary and tertiary services.

Secondary care includes services that are more sophisticated and complicated than those defined within primary care. As Barton says, "secondary care…signals a higher level of intensity, often over a longer period of time, than event-specific primary care" (2). It is at the level of secondary care that most physician specialists work. For example, here are specialists such as ophthalmologists, gastroenterologists, orthopedists, cardiologists, urologists and so on. As with primary care, any one of these specialties is not exclusively defined within secondary care; there may be some overlap of both primary care and tertiary care in the services that they provide. For example, a cardiologist may provide diagnosis at a basic level when a heart condition is suspected (primary care) and may also be part of a surgical team in open heart surgery (tertiary care).

Tertiary care then is a level at which diagnoses and interventions are yet more sophisticated and deal with more complicated surgical and other procedures. This level of care usually addresses complex conditions and procedurally intensive inpatient care. Tertiary care is typically offered in an academic medical center or a large community hospital where numbers of medical specialists team up to perform procedures such as transplants, open heart surgery, neurosurgery, and specialized diagnostic procedures, such as positron emission tomography (PET).

While the term "tertiary care" has been used to describe the highest technologic level of care available, ongoing medical advances have taken us beyond the realm of our historical definition of tertiary care. With the advances that medicine has made possible in the past several years, the ability and skills to perform even more highly complex procedures in very complicated cases have also advanced. The categorization of "quaternary care" has been designated as a level of care in which procedures such as multiple organ transplants, specialized burn units, very delicate procedures in neurology, and other such specialized services are performed.

3.2.4 Other Categorizations of Healthcare Service Levels

Healthcare providers are further categorized based on the types and needs of the patients they are serving. Again, these further subdivisions do not necessarily apply exclusively — there may be some overlap with the four hierarchical categorizations discussed above. For example, within long-term nursing care, we may find both primary care and some secondary care services offered.

3.2.4.1   Ambulatory Care

By contrast to the acute inpatient setting in which the patient is admitted and stays overnight for one or more days, in the ambulatory care setting, the patient is able to enter and leave on the same day. Ambulatory care is that which is provided in outpatient surgery and diagnostic centers, walk-in clinics, physician offices, and other such venues. Ambulatory care went through swift and dramatic growth in the mid- to late 1980s and into the 1990s and has become a major sector in the provision of healthcare.

Ambulatory care was extensively expanded during the latter part of the 1980s and into the 1990s due to the convergence of several changing factors. First, with the passage of the prospective payment system in 1983, the diagnosis-related group payment structure was put in place to control the level of reimbursement that Medicare (and later, other payers) paid to hospitals for inpatient acute care. Hospitals quickly looked for other venues in which they could provide care; they looked for ways to reduce inpatient admissions for those services for which there was a lowered reimbursement — they found ambulatory care ready and waiting. Endoscopy and the laser had been developed and made minimally invasive surgery possible. It thereby offered the opportunity for many surgeries to transition from the inpatient setting to the outpatient setting. Additionally, ambulatory care had not yet come under the controlled reimbursement of the prospective payment system. Factors such as these created the perfect environment in which ambulatory care could grow and thrive. It was not until about a decade later that the Centers for Medicare and Medicaid Services (CMS) adopted a structure of ambulatory payment

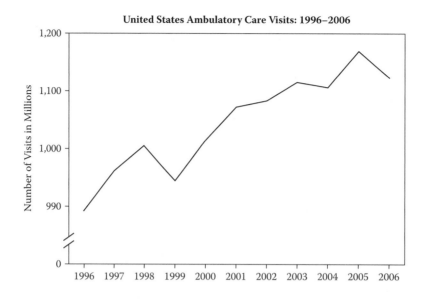

Figure 3.3   U.S. ambulatory care visits: 1996–2006. Number of ambulance ser-vices: 813; number of ambulatory surgery centers: 1,040. Source: Health Forum, American Hospital Association. "AHA Hospital Statistics." Health Forum LLC. 2008 Edition. "From 1996–2006, the number of ambulatory care visits overall increased by 26 percent. Patients in the United States made an estimated 1.1 billion visits to physician offices and hospital OPDs and EDs, a rate of 381.9 visits per 100 persons annually." Source: S. M. Schappert and E. A. Rechtsteiner. Ambulatory medical care utilization estimates for 2006. National Health Statistics Reports, no. 8. Hyattsville, MD. National Center for Health Statistics, 2008. http://www.cdc.gov/nchs/data/nhsr/nhsr008.pdf

groups (APGs) in order to control reimbursements for ambulatory care. This, then, was a decade of substantial expansion of ambulatory care centers.

Despite the reimbursement controls implemented by the Centers for Medicare and Medicaid Services, ambulatory care has continued to grow. From 1996 to 2006, the number of ambulatory care visits overall increased by 26%, and patients in the United States made an estimated 1.1 billion visits to physician offices and hospital Outpatient Department (OPD) and Emergency Departments (ED), a rate of 381.9 visits per 100 persons annually (4) (Figure 3.3).

As outlined above, ambulatory care is provided in a number of settings, including physician offices, clinics, hospital OPDs, EDs, freestanding ambu-latory care centers or urgent care centers, surgicenters, and the more recent phenomenon of mini-clinics. Let us define a couple of these:

■ Surgicenters: Surgicenters are typically freestanding centers dedicated to surgical procedures that can be performed on an ambulatory basis. Patients do not have overnight stays in surgicenters; they are admitted and discharged on the same day of service.

■ OPDs: Hospital OPDs provide diagnostic capabilities that may not be offered in the physician office (e.g., laboratory tests, radiology, CT scans, MRI and other such services). They may also provide capacity for outpatient surgery and treatment, such as kidney dialysis, chemotherapy, and radiation therapy.

■ Urgent care centers: Urgent care centers, also known as ambulatory care centers, may be
    1. freestanding under private ownership,
    2. freestanding off-campus from a hospital or health system owner,
    3. situated on a hospital campus.

These centers are typically open for longer hours than physician offices, are equipped to perform basic radiology and laboratory procedures, and can perform minor surgical procedures that might otherwise be performed in an ED. Urgent care centers offer convenience to the public who may not have to travel a distance to get to the center and who do not have to go through the more complicated processing and long waits that are typical of hospital ED visits.

■ Mini-clinics: Mini-clinics are a more recent development and have "popped up" in pharmacies and grocery stores across the country. These clinics are generally staffed by a nurse practitioner, are open during convenient hours for people coming into the retail store, and provide a list of specific services that they provide and the related fees they charge for those services. Their services meet basic needs for people with colds, flu, and other common ailments. Many also provide physicals for students who require these to participate in school athletic programs. Charges may be in the range of $45 to $60, appointments are typically not required and visits may take about 15 minutes.

■ Public health clinics: While we cover public health more extensively later in this book, it is appropriate to mention here that public health clinics also provide an essential range of basic health services for persons who are indigent or who otherwise lack access to care. While some public health clinics provide a full range of primary care services, others limit their services to maternal and child care, to immunizations, and/or to screening. These clinics are funded by federal, state, and local tax-based funds, and most utilize a sliding-fee schedule to charge the patient a portion of the established fee based on that person's income. Similar clinics are also operated by some faith-based groups. These are primarily financed by faith-based organizations and through charges to Medicare and Medicaid and in part through sliding-fee schedules related to the patient's financial resources.

3.2.4.2 Subacute Care

Subacute care falls between the acute and long-term levels of care. At the subacute level, patients receive care that helps facilitate their recovery from major injury or an episode of illness (e.g., stroke). "Subacute care is a mix of rehabilitation and convalescent services that requires 10 to 100 days of care. It is a level and duration of care inappropriate to either acute care hospitals or to most skilled nursing facilities" (5). Subacute units will be found primarily in hospitals and or skilled nursing care facilities that create units designed for the level of nursing services required by the sub-acute care patient. In some cases, nursing homes have converted beds to subacute care, and in other instances, hospitals have modified or built inpatient units to accommodate the subacute level of service. The care provided in a subacute unit may include nursing intensive services such as intubation and/or ventilator support.

3.2.4.3 Long-Term Care

While long-term care may technically refer to any care that requires a duration of 30 days or more, it is more typically perceived in a narrower definition as being what we know as "nursing home" care, which is dominantly used by the elderly and to a lesser extent by persons with disabilities that impede their performance of certain "activities of daily living" (e.g., dressing, feeding themselves, toileting, etc.). As Sultz and Young put it: "The age, diagnosis, and ability to perform personal self-care and the sites of care delivery vary widely for recipients of long-term care" (5). The following discusses those sites of care delivery.

3.2.4.3.1 Nursing Care Facilities

Long-term nursing care facilities may offer several levels of care, including subacute care (discussed above), skilled nursing care and intermediate care. Under the Medicare program, nursing facility services are distinguished and reimbursed based on the level of care the residents require as measured by their medical condition and their capacity to perform activities of daily living. The Medicare classification system utilizes the Resource Utilization

Groups, Version III (RUDIII) to designate the level of care that a resident receives and the reimbursement that is provided for that care. The RUGIII, Version III establishes a clinical hierarchy among various patient needs, such as rehabilitation, extensive services, behavior problems, and cognition, and does so with a sublevel or second level in which activities of daily living are measured (e.g., feeding, clothing, bathing, toileting).

Unlike acute care hospitals, most nursing facilities in the United States are owned by proprietary organizations. Many are owned by for-profit companies that own multiple facilities in a region or throughout the country, others are owned privately by church-based organizations and still others are owned by healthcare systems or by local governments. Currently, there are about 18,000 nursing homes in the United States offering a total of 1.9 million beds that are 87% occupied with 1.6 million residents (6) (Table 3.3).

Charges for care in nursing homes are reported on a monthly basis. Table 3.4 provides data from the Centers for Disease Control and Prevention's National Center for Health Statistics and reflects that the typical

Table 3.3 U.S. Nursing Homes Overall Statistics: 2004

Number of Nursing Homes	16,100
Number of Nursing Home Beds	1,730,000
Number of Current Residents	1,492,200
Occupancy Rate	86.3%
Average Length of Stay (current resident)	892 days

Source: National Center for Health Statistics. Health, United States, 2007: With Chartbook on Trends in the Health of Americans." Table 117. Hyattsville, MD: National Center for Health Statistics, 2007.

Table 3.4 Average Monthly Charges for Nursing Home Care: 1985–2004

Year	Average Monthly Charges ($)
1985	1,508
1995	3,132
1997	3,638
1999	3,531
2004	5,690

Source: National Center for Health Statistics. *Health, United States, 2007, With Chartbook on Trends in the Health of Americans.* Table 132. Hyattsville, MD: National Center for Health Statistics, 2007.

monthly charge in the United States in 2007 was $5,690 for the average patient (6). However, charges may be more or less based on ownership, Medicare certification, bed size and geographic region (see Table 3.4).

The average age of nursing residents has gone up over the past decades. In 2004, the National Center for Health Statistics reported that of every 1000 persons between 65 and 74 years old, 9.4 were in nursing facilities; of those between 75 and 84 years old, 36.1 were in nursing homes; and for every 1000 persons aged 85 years or older, 138.7 lived in such facilities. These rates are down from 10.8, 43.0, and 182.5, respectively, just 5 years before, in 1999 (6) (Table 3.5).

Nursing facility revenues come from three major sources: self-pay patients, Medicare and Medicaid. Medicaid is by far the largest source of revenue for nursing facilities, providing approximately 46% of the total (7) (Figure 3.4). When individuals are admitted to nursing homes, if they have the financial means and do not meet the poverty guidelines of Medicaid, they will "spend down" their personal wealth in covering the cost of care. Once that personal wealth is depleted to Medicaid eligibility levels, the patients may be enrolled in Medicaid, which pays for the cost of long-term care from that point forward.

There has been controversy over this policy of impoverishment for the elderly in order for them to qualify for Medicaid coverage for long-term care. State laws are strict on the transfer of money and assets from potential or actual nursing facility residents to family or friends in order to meet the financial qualification levels to enroll in Medicaid. The principle under which the states operate is that the taxpayers should not have to cover the cost of care for someone who has the financial ability to pay for his or her

Table 3.5 Nursing Facility Residents as Portion of the Total Population: 1999 and 2004

Age	Residents per 1,000 Population					
	1999			2004		
	All	Male	Female	All	Male	Female
65-74 years	10.8	10.3	11.2	9.4	8.9	9.8
75-84 years	43.0	30.8	51.2	36.1	27.0	42.3
85 years and over	182.5	116.5	210.5	138.7	80.0	165.2

Source: National Center for Health Statistics. *Health, United States, 2007: With Chartbook on Trends in the Health of Americans.* Table 104. Hyattsville, MD: National Center for Health Statistics, 2007.

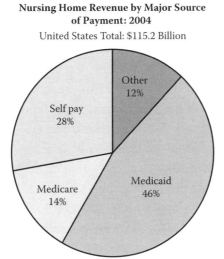

**Nursing Home Revenue by Major Source
of Payment: 2004**
United States Total: $115.2 Billion

Other 12%
Self pay 28%
Medicare 14%
Medicaid 46%

Figure 3.4 Nursing home revenue by major source of payment: 2004. Sources: C. Smith, C. Cowan, S. Heffler, A. Catlin, and the National Health Accounts Team, 2006. *Health Affairs.* 25(1), 186–196; California Office of Statewide Health Planning and Development, long term care annual financial data, 2004, and hospital financial data estimates, 2004.

care. In other words, taxpayers should not have to bear the financial burden of long-term care only to have the individual leave an estate to his or her family — an estate made possible because taxpayers would have paid the cost of care.

3.2.4.3.2   Assisted Living

Within the classification of long-term care are also assisted living facilities. With the aging of the population and the increasing longevity of the older population, along with their improving financial status and the fact that they are staying healthy longer, the demand for accommodations offering supportive care, rather than inpatient nursing care, has grown. As the older population ages and experiences a gradually diminishing physical capacity, many want to relinquish their individual homes and move into an environment in which meals and support services are provided, transportation is available, and companionship is at hand. The growth of assisted living facilities has, as a result, been dynamic since the turn of the twenty-first century.

In some cases, developers and owners of long-term care services form continuing care retirement communities (CCRCs), which serve the needs of individuals at whatever their physical status might be as they age. CCRCs typically offer a full range of housing from independent living in houses or apartments to assisted living to skilled nursing or the nursing care facility. Many also offer Alzheimer's disease and other specialty care units. With the availability of this range of services, a resident may move into whatever level of care he or she needs when it is needed. In other words, once individuals move into a CCRC, they are guaranteed that, as their health deteriorates or should they need increased medical and personal support on a short-term basis, the facility will provide the level required. The advantage of this to the resident is that he or she does not need to find a new place to live as his or her physical condition changes. Human beings tend to become increasingly sensitive to place with advancing age. The CCRC offers the opportunity to stay in place rather than making a dramatic change of place to find the level of care needed. Most CCRCs are fully private pay facilities and do not accept Medicaid reimbursement.

3.2.4.4   Home Health Care

Home healthcare is generally organized by a voluntary community organization or a hospital. Agencies providing home healthcare send caregivers into the home of the patients. Those caregivers may be registered or licensed practical nurses, aides, therapists, or others who assist the patients with their medical needs, such as monitoring blood pressure and medications and changing bandages; in physical, occupational, and speech therapy; and in supportive areas such as meal preparation, household chores, transportation, and so on. Under Medicare, home health agencies may be certified for reimbursement, and once certified they are termed a certified home health service. Patients who are covered by Medicare for payment of their home healthcare must meet three requirements: (1) they must be homebound; (2) a plan of treatment is required to be both prepared and reviewed periodically by a physician; and (3) the patients must require periodic or part-time skilled nursing and/or rehabilitation therapies.

Home health agencies may be owned by hospitals, a visiting nurse association, a for-profit proprietary company, a community-based organization, or other types of entity. The number of home healthcare agencies is on a constant rise (see Figure 3.5), and expenditures for home health services have grown dramatically since the late 1990s. Those expenditures dipped significantly in the mid-1990s due to a high-profile case of fraudulent billing. With the solution of that case, the country has again embraced home health as a more inexpensive and sensitive way to deliver medical care (see Figure 3.6).

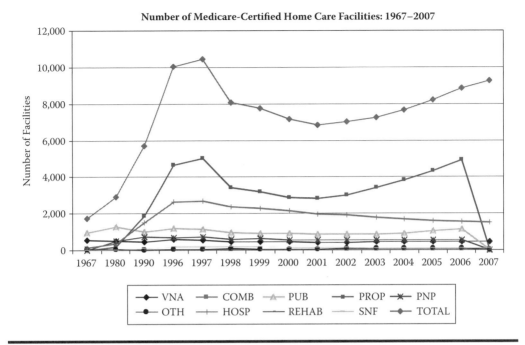

Figure 3.5   Number of Medicare-certified home care facilities: 1967–2007. Data source: Centers for Medicare and Medicaid Services (CMS), Center for Information Systems, Health Standards and Quality Bureau (2006 data obtained in February 2007). Definitions source: National Association for Home Care and Hospice. "Basic Statistics About Home Care," 2008. Accessed September 9, 2008. http://www.nahc. org/facts/08HC_Stats.pdf. VNA: Visiting nurse associations are freestanding, voluntary, nonprofit organizations governed by a board of directors and usually financed by tax-deductible contributions as well as by earnings. COMB: Combination agencies are combined government and voluntary agencies. These agencies are sometimes included with counts for VNAs. PUB: Public agencies are government agencies operated by a state, county, city, or other unit of local government having a major responsibility for preventing disease and for community health education. PROP: Proprietary agencies are freestanding, for-profit home care agencies. PNP: Private not-for-profit agencies are freestanding and privately developed, governed, and owned nonprofit home care agencies. These agencies were not counted separately before 1980. OTH: Other freestanding agencies that do not fit one of the categories for freestanding agencies listed above. HOSP: Hospital-based agencies are operating units or departments of a hospital. Agencies that have working arrangements with a hospital, or perhaps are even owned by a hospital but operated as separate entities, are classified as freestanding agencies under one of the categories listed above. REHAB: refers to agencies based in rehabilitation facilities. SNF: Refers to agencies based in skilled nursing facilities.

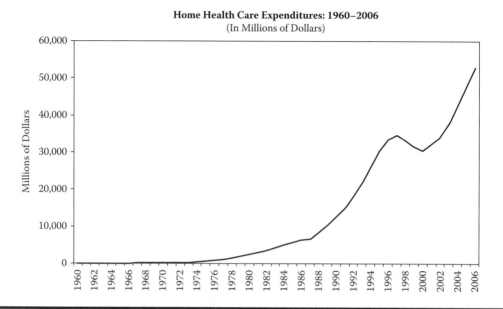

Home Health Care Expenditures: 1960–2006
(In Millions of Dollars)

Figure 3.6   Home healthcare expenditures: 1960–2006. Source: Centers for Medicaid and Medicare Services. "National Health Expenditures by type of service and source of funds, CY 1960–2006." National Health Expenditure Historical Data. Accessed September 2008. http://www.cms.hhs.gov/NationalHealthExpendData/02_NationalHealthAccountsHistorical.asp#TopOfPage

3.2.4.5   Hospice care

Hospice care is a relatively recent phenomenon in healthcare. Its growth was spurred by legislation passed in 1982 that provided Medicare coverage for hospice care. This legislation required hospitals to seek out patients' wishes relative to advanced directives, such as DNR (do not resuscitate) options, and to encourage them to appoint someone with power of attorney to make decisions for them in a situation in which they cannot make decisions for themselves.

The most common measure by which a patient is admitted into hospice care is that he or she is terminally ill and has a life expectancy of up to 6 months. While in hospice care, the patient receives palliative care, which is care that addresses pain management and other physical interventions to provide for the patient's comfort during the last months, weeks, or days of life. It is care that attempts to "relieve the symptoms of a disease rather than attempting to cure the disease" (5). The patient in hospice care is the person who does not want aggressive medical treatment and who has decided that it is more personally desirable to forego aggressive and often invasive, expensive treatment in favor of a potentially shorter life with more quality and peace away from the intensiveness of sophisticated medical interventions that might otherwise be used. Care is typically provided by a multidisciplinary team consisting of physicians, nurses, counselors, psychologists, social workers, and therapists. Typically, all medical supplies and drugs, as well as the required professional nursing and supportive services, are financially covered 100% by Medicare and other payers. Hospice supports not only the terminally ill patient but also the family in their bereavement following the death of the patient.

The number of hospice facilities and cost of hospice care have increased steadily over the past 5 years (Figure 3.7). Figure 3.8 indicates that Medicare and Medicaid expenditures for hospice care have increased substantially since 2000 (8).

3.2.4.6   Respite and Day Care

Respite and adult day care are "opposite sides of the same coin." Adult day care is a service in which an elderly person, or someone whose physical condition requires continuous care, is cared for outside the home in a group

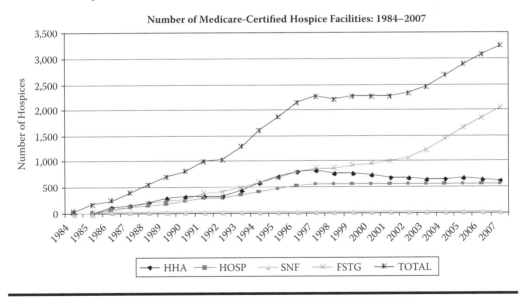

Figure 3.7   Number of Medicare-certified hospice facilities: 1984–2007. Source: Hospice Association of America. "Hospice Facts and Statistics," March 2008. Accessed September 2008. http://www.nahc.org/facts/HospiceStats08.pdf In 2007, of the 3,257 Medicare-certified hospices, 2,050 were freestanding (FSTG), 627 were home health agency based (HHA), 562 were hospital based (HOSP), and 18 were skilled nursing facility based (SNF). There are also an estimated 200 volunteer agencies that are not Medicare certified.

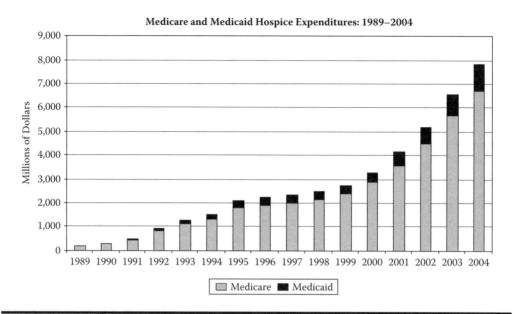

Figure 3.8   Medicare and Medicaid hospice expenditures: 1989–2004. Source: Hospice Association of America. "Hospice Facts and Statistics," March 2008. Accessed September 2008. http://www.nahc.org/facts/HospiceStats08.pdf Data obtained from Centers for Medicare and Medicaid Services. "CMS-64 Quarterly Expense Report" (Form CMS-64, updated March 2008). www.cms.gov. Accessed September 2008. Note: FY 1996 totals exclude data for Florida and Hawaii. FY 1997 totals exclude data for Hawaii. FY 1999 and FY 2000 totals exclude Medicaid SCHIP.

setting during the work day or any other scheduled period. In a typical scenario, the person who is "dropped off" at the day care center is provided supportive assistance while the full-time caregiver goes to work. Respite care, on the other hand, is provided in order to support the caregiver for whom the demands of constant care giving can be stressful and very time consuming. Respite care provides a setting in which the one being cared for can stay in a safe supportive place while the caregiver has time to perform errands or to travel or "get away" for several days or a week. Adult day care services are typically tied to a nursing facility and, in some cases, to a community senior center. Respite care, because it is overnight care, is typically a service offered by a nursing facility.

3.2.4.7   Rehabilitation

Rehabilitation services provide physical, occupational, and speech therapies for patients who have suffered an illness or injury that leaves them with some level of physical disability. "Rehabilitation...provides specialized care to assist patients in achieving optimal physical, mental and social functioning after resolution of an illness or injury" (5).

While there are a number of hospital-based inpatient rehabilitation units throughout the country, rehabilitation is more generally provided on an outpatient basis and is included in the services that nursing care facilities provide to patients. In outpatient rehabilitation facilities, a physiatrist is the clinical specialist physician who provides medically licensed service and leadership to the organization, and he or she is supported by physical, occupational and speech therapists as well as social workers and counselors.

Currently, there are 198 rehabilitation hospitals in the United States, and they offer 15,106 inpatient beds for more than a quarter of a million admissions each year (9) (Table 3.6).

3.2.4.8   Emergency Services

Emergency services (EMS) are part of healthcare delivery in rural and urban areas across the country, and they are also a key part of the fabric of healthcare. Their organization varies from a volunteer model to a corporate model. Their locus also varies. Emergency services are frequently housed with other community services, such as a fire department, and in yet other instances they are situated within the campus of hospitals and medical centers. Their staffing may also be structured differently. Volunteer emergency services often do not have paramedics and EMTs (emergency medical technicians) on-site waiting for a call. Instead, volunteers stay "at the ready" and respond to the call to get to the emergency vehicles immediately. In other instances, full-time, round-the-clock paid personnel staff the emergency service.

Table 3.6 Rehabilitation Hospitals in the United States: 2007

	United States	Rehabilitation Hospitals
Hospitals	5,747	198
Beds	947,412	15,106
Admissions	37,188,775	270,245
Inpatient Days	238,203,381	3,814,271
Emergency Outpatient Visits	122,628,450	8,916
Total Outpatient Visits	690,425,395	6,347,934

Source: Health Forum, American Hospital Association. "AHA Hospital Statistics." Chicago: Health Forum LLC, 2008.

Staffing may also vary in the level of training required. Frequently, paramedics are not available or assigned to ride to the scene of an emergency unless the dispatcher notes that the extent of illness or injury requires the more highly trained professional.

3.2.4.9   Mental Health and Substance Abuse

Healthcare provider organizations that provide mental healthcare are typically either psychiatric facilities or substance abuse facilities. Mental healthcare may be provided on either an inpatient or an outpatient basis. The dramatic improvements in psychotropic drugs of the past several decades have provided the opportunity for mental healthcare to move primarily to an outpatient setting.

3.3   Summary

This chapter has provided the descriptions and essential characteristics of the various entities through which healthcare is delivered in the United States. With the exception of physician practices, these are the entities that play central roles in healthcare delivery. There are several other venues that support healthcare, including alternative and holistic medicine centers, chiropractic and podiatric care, vision care centers, and others. These are of significant benefit to many consumers, and many of their services are included under third-party payer arrangements. While the latter are not discussed in this book, they certainly merit acknowledgment and it should be recognized that they are growing in both number and volume of service in the United States.

References

1. A. R. Kovner and J. R. Knickman, 2008. *Jonas and Kovner's Health Care Delivery in the United States*, 9th Edition. Springer: New York, p. 213.
2. P. L. Barton, 2004. *Understanding the U.S. Health Services System*. Health Administration Press, Ann Arbor, MI, p. 353.
3. Institute of Medicine, 1995. In: P. L. Barton, p. 343.
4. S. M. Schappert and E. A. Rechtsteiner, 2008. "Ambulatory Medical Care Utilization Estimates for 2006. National Health Statistics Reports, No. 8." National Center for Health Statistics, Hyattsville, MD. Accessed November 2008. Available at: http://www.cdc.gov/nchs/data/nhsr/nhsr008.pdf

5. H. A. Sultz and K. M. Young, 2009. *Health Care USA*. Jones and Bartlett Publishers, Sudbury, MA, pp. 86, 98, and 302.

6. National Center for Health Statistics, 2007. "Health, United States, 2007, With Chartbook on Trends in the Health of Americans." National Center for Health Statistics, Hyattsville, MD, Table 117.

7. C. Smith, C. Cowan, S. Heffler, A. Catlin, and the National Accounts Team, 2006. "California Office of Statewide Planning and Development, Long Term Care Annual Financial Data, 2004, and Hospital Financial Data Estimates." *Health Affairs*, 25(1), 186–196.

8. Hospice Association of America, 2008. "Hospice Facts and Statistics." Accessed September 2008. Available at: http://www.nahc.org/facts/HospiceStats08.pdf

9. Health Forum, American Hospital Association, 2008. *AHA Hospital Statistics 2008 Edition*. Health Forum, LLC, Chicago, IL.

Websites

Association of American Medical Colleges (AAMC): http://www.aamc.org
Centers for Medicaid and Medicare Services (CMS): http://www.cms.hhs.gov
Hospice Association of America (HAA): http://www.nahc.org/hospice/
National Association for Home Care and Hospice (NAHC): http://www.nahc.org
National Center for Health Statistics (NCHS): http://www.cdc.gov/nchs/
United States Department of Veterans Affairs (VA): http://www.va.gov

Chapter 4

Structure of Healthcare Delivery

4.1 Introduction

In the last chapter, we discussed the various components or types of healthcare providers. Although they were described individually, they also comprise the "continuum of care." The continuum of care includes all the different types of providers of care that a patient might need to access as he or she goes through a diagnostic and treatment process. For example, the patient who has had a stroke may initially access care through the emergency department, from which he or she is then moved to an intensive care unit in the hospital, then to a subacute unit, then to a rehabilitation facility, and perhaps to home to be cared for by home health providers. Each of these provider entities may be under different ownership and corporate structures, but each is inextricably linked from the patient's perspective. However, that link is one-sided. Too often, these providers of care are not organizationally linked and full information does not flow from one to another. As the patient moves through the continuum, he or she must create a new relationship with each provider, including new paperwork, new insurance approvals, and new protocols of care. Each is meant to build on the work of the previous provider, but lacking electronic communication, often the transition of care and of information among providers is fraught with error and miscommunication.

In this chapter, we discuss the linkages, and lack thereof, among the various providers of care. First, we discuss the organizational structures under which providers function, we expand on defining distinctions among providers within the classifications that were addressed in chapter 3, and we discuss their interdependencies and the challenges of those interdependencies.

4.2 Hospital Classifications

In chapter 3, we discussed classification of healthcare providers based on the services they provide. All the provider organizations identified in chapter 3 may also be classified in a number of other ways, including classification by (1) ownership, (2) tax status, and (3) geographic location.

Each has its own unique impact on the operation of the hospital, and all apply for each hospital. For example, a hospital owned by a faith-based group may be tax-exempt, it may be situated in a rural area, and it may be a general acute care hospital. We discuss each in turn.

4.2.1 Ownership

One term that is often used to describe healthcare organizations is "private," the opposite of which is "public" when describing organizations in the health sector and in other sectors of the economy. Most hospitals and organizational providers of care, with the exception of those operated by governmental entities such as the Veterans Administration (VA), Indian Health Services (IHS), county and municipal hospitals (e.g., Grady Hospital in Atlanta, Stroger Hospital in Chicago), and prison hospitals, are considered private hospitals. Public hospitals are organized and operated under the authority of a government entity.

4.2.1.1 Private Healthcare Entities

Private healthcare entities are any that are not owned by the public body. *Private* in this classification means that they are owned and operated under the auspices of a defined group. They may be organized and operated under the auspices of a community. Having been founded by community leaders (such as a school might be established), the assets are owned by that community. An initial board of directors is appointed to the healthcare organization, and that board operates continuously. Members have term limits, and when a member's term expires, he or she is replaced by Board selection of new members from the community.

Some private hospitals are owned by *for-profit corporations*. These corporations may be owned by a group of private individuals or formed as public corporations, with their stock trading on a public stock exchange.

Many private healthcare organizations are *church-related organizations*. Historically, a number of faith-based organizations developed hospitals and clinics to care for persons in a locality for which the organization determined that there were a need and an opportunity to serve both the spiritual and physical needs of their faithful. The founding of hospitals by faith-based groups, such as the Baptists, Methodists, Lutherans, Presbyterians, Jews, and Catholics, was inspired not only by the needs of their members but also by the needs arising out of the illness of individuals who were made particularly vulnerable by that illness and out of the needs of populations who had no access to medical services. Today, most of those faith-based organizations maintain their original mission of caring for the needy and for their members. They do not limit their care to persons of their religious beliefs, and they operate competitively beside other nonprofit and for-profit health systems. About 14% of the hospitals in the United States are owned by faith-based organizations (Figure 4.1).

4.2.1.2   Community and Voluntary Providers of Care

Hospitals and other healthcare providers are frequently characterized by the terms "community" and/or "voluntary" hospital. The term *community hospital* may be used for those hospitals that are founded and owned by a local community, by a religious sect, or by a for-profit company. It is broadly applied to those hospitals that serve the locality in which they operate and is typically used in contrast to the categorization of other hospitals as academic medical centers or teaching hospitals.

The healthcare entity that is characterized as *voluntary* is one that has been founded by a volunteer effort in the community. This is typically applied to nonprofit hospitals that are owned by a faith-based organization or by a community (not as a public hospital as described below).

4.2.1.3   Government/Public Hospitals and Clinics

Government/public hospitals and clinics are those that are operated by federal, state, or local governments. Public hospitals are organized and operated

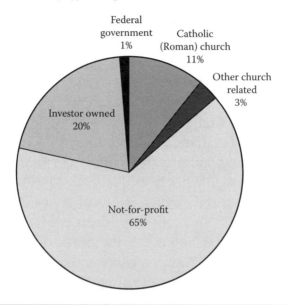

**Figure 4.1   Multihospital healthcare systems by type of organizational control.
Source: Health Forum, American Hospital Association.** *AHA Hospital Statistics.*
Chicago: Health Forum LLC, 2008.

under the authority of the respective government entity. Any shortfalls in
their financial operations are paid with taxpayer dollars. Many local public
hospitals originated as places for indigents whose care was the responsibility
of the local government. They have evolved over time to state-of-the-art tertiary organizations. While they continue to serve primarily indigent persons
and those on Medicaid, many of them have developed top-rated emergency
departments and trauma centers and other specialized services.

Other public hospitals and medical services are those owned by the
VA, which operates them for retired members of the military. The VA fully
finances the medical care of those discharged individuals. One limitation on
retired military individuals is that, depending on where they live, they may
have limited geographical access to their VA hospital. Overall, the VA provides
696 outpatient clinics, 174 hospitals, and 250 veterans' centers (Table 4.1).

Government or publicly owned providers of care are also found on
Indian reservations where the IHS spends over $3 billion annually on
healthcare services under treaties entered into between native tribes and
Alaska Eskimos and the U.S. government. These treaties date back to the
early founding of the country. The 12 IHS area offices administer 155 IHS-

Table 4.1 Veterans Affairs Clinics, Hospitals and Centers: 2008

Medical Facility	*Number of Facilities*
Outpatient Clinic	696
Hospitals	174
Veterans' Centers	250

Source: United States Department of Veterans Affairs. "Facilities Locator and Directory.". Updated March 2008. On-line source (accessed September 2008). http://www1.va.gov/directory/guide/rpt_fac_list.cfm

operated and tribally operated healthcare units. The facilities they provide are primarily health clinics. A limited number of hospitals (Figure 4.2) are provided on Indian reservations and are supported through the IHS as well.

4.2.2 Tax Status: Taxed or Tax-Exempt

Healthcare organizations function under a number of corporate and tax structures. Some are established as for-profit entities, others as not-for-profit

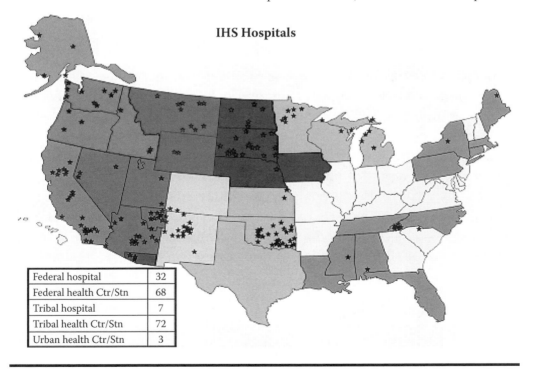

Federal hospital	32
Federal health Ctr/Stn	68
Tribal hospital	7
Tribal health Ctr/Stn	72
Urban health Ctr/Stn	3

Figure 4.2 IHS Hospitals in the U.S. Source: U.S. Dept. of Health and Human Services (IHS). 2008. Accessed October 2008. Available at http://www.ihs.gov/ NonMedicalPrograms/chs/index.cfm?module=chs_program_directory.

entities; most not-for-profit healthcare provider organizations are tax-exempt, while for-profit entities pay federal, state, and local taxes unless they are given a specific tax exemption by the respective level of government under which they operate (e.g., some may be exempt from paying property taxes for a period as an inducement to locate in a given municipality). "Tax exemption is often also considered as a subsidy for the costs federal or local government would otherwise incur to provide important but costly health services" (1). This is also called "community benefit." In return for this sub-sidy, the tax-exempt entity is expected to provide free services to the com-munity. This is callled "community benefit." Community benefit is typically comprised of free care for indigents, community education programs in prevention (e.g., smoking cessation), and screening clinics.

There is no set standard for the financial levels at which a community benefit should be established. Some states are entertaining proposals for tax-exempt hospitals to provide free services equal to 2% of their revenue; other states are seeking levels of up to 6%–7% of revenues. While there is no consensus on a standard yet, the IRS has issued a new Schedule H of the 990 Form that nonprofits are required to complete and submit. This sched-ule requires hospitals to fully disclose their community benefits for tax years beginning in 2009. Bad debts and Medicare discounts are not eligible for consideration as community benefits (2).

As local governments face revenue shortfalls and increasing demand for tax revenues to support infrastructure and public services, they will con-tinue to examine the value they receive from their local nonprofit hospi-tal. They will question whether or not the community benefit provided by the nonprofit hospital(s) adequately meets the value of foregone taxes. For example, a 2007 report of hospital values in Cook County, Illinois, indicated that if all the tax-exempt hospitals in the county paid property taxes, the value would be between $238 and $241 million (3). In pressing financial circumstances, it is compelling for local governments to review the commu-nity service value they are getting for the tax exemptions they provide.

4.2.2.1   Not-for-Profit

Not-for-profit hospitals and health systems operate under the financial prin-ciple that no net revenue or profit is paid to individuals or organizations based on investment in, or ownership of, the nonprofit organization. In other words, the nonprofit may record a positive bottom line on its income and expense statement, but the amounts reflected on that bottom line are retained and reinvested in the organization; they are not paid out as investment income. There is no individual investment ownership of the nonprofit.

However, the nonprofit healthcare provider does employ management, professional, and support and clinical staff to carry out the duties and tasks required to run a complicated organization. These staff members include everyone from the president/CEO to doctors, nurses, technologists, therapists, pharmacists, dietitians, maintenance, and office personnel. Each of them is paid what are typically competitive salaries.

Some individuals have the perception that if a hospital or any other medical provider is established as a nonprofit, it must not make profit. The nonprofit establishes charges for services that are competitive with other providers in the area and structures its budget to achieve a profit after all expenses are paid or accounted for.

In some cases, nonprofit healthcare systems may own a for-profit entity, such as a managed care organization or one in which real estate is held and rented out on a for-profit basis until that real estate is needed for health service expansion. In these cases, the subsidiary for-profit company is required to pay taxes on net revenues or profit.

4.2.2.2 For-Profit

For-profit hospitals have existed in the United States for decades. In the early history of the United States, many hospitals were founded and owned by physicians. The origin of the for-profit multihospital corporation dates back to the 1960s when several companies such as Hospital Corporation of America (known today as "The Hospital Company") were founded. Entrepreneurial investors found fertile ground primarily in the South, where many small community hospitals were owned by physicians or by those small towns. The sale of the community-owned local hospital was particularly attractive in light of its equity value and its operations on the one hand and because of the demands upon local governments for monies to invest in other community services, such as improved schools and jails. These investment dollars, earned through the sale of the community's hospital to a for-profit hospital operator provided the funds for other essential community services while maintaining the hospital in the community. With the advent of Medicare and Medicaid and the proliferation of commercial health insurance through employer funding, and in a time when hospital bills were paid without question by these organizations, hospitals had strong equity value and provided opportunity for profitability — both attractive characteristics to the investor.

Today there are a number of for-profit hospital companies, both large and small. They own varying number of hospitals, but, typically, those hospitals are geographically dispersed and not networked or fully integrated for the sharing of patient and financial or other operational information. They operate under the same rules and regulations of nonprofit hospitals; however, a key purpose of their ownership is that they return a profit to investors. Often they are criticized for not providing the level of charity or indigent care as do nonprofit hospitals. Yet, overall, they report data indicating that they participate substantially in supporting indigent care in their communities; despite the fact that they do not hold tax exemption.

4.2.3 Geography

Hospitals may also be classified as urban or rural. Each of these classifications has implications for the way in which Medicare reimbursement is calculated. In part, that calculation looks at the different costs of urban and rural operations. Many rural hospitals are smaller facilities and do not have the revenue-generating capacity of their urban counterparts, particularly in the more lucrative specialty services such as cardiology and orthopedics. As small hospitals, highly dependent on Medicare and Medicaid, many of these hospitals need proportionately higher reimbursement in order to remain operational. Under the category of "critical-access hospital" (CAH), their reimbursement is determined based on their expenses rather than on a predetermined diagnosis-related group reimbursement level. There are two geographic classifications of hospitals: urban and rural.

■ Urban: Hospitals classified as urban hospitals are those that are located in a metropolitan statistical area of 50,000 or larger population.
■ Rural: Rural hospitals are those that are not located in a metropolitan statistical area. The importance of this distinction is relevant in that it is one of the factors considered in computing reimbursement. Certain rural hospitals are designated as CAHs under Medicare. Because these facilities are deemed to provide a critical source of access to care for the residents of the area in which they are located and based on the premise that there is no other access point to inpatient medical care in

the area, these hospitals are reimbursed by Medicare on a cost-based system rather than on a prospective payment or diagnosis-related group basis. This designation was established under the 1997 Balanced Budget Act, which calls for specific conditions under which the designation may be used. For example, the hospital may be no larger than 25 inpatient beds, may have no more than a 96-hour average length of stay, and may not have distinct service units such as orthopedics and psychiatry. By the end of 2007, 1292 rural hospitals were designated as CAHs (see Figure 4.3).

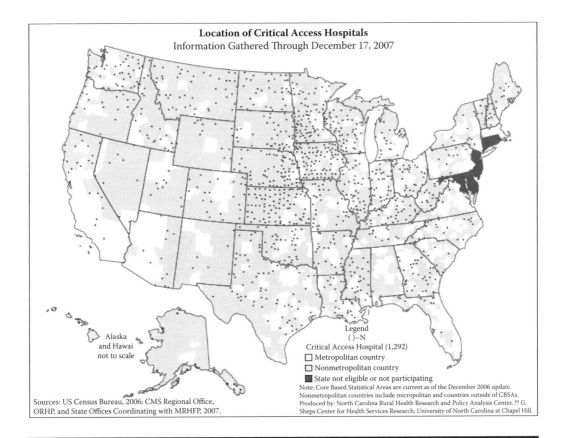

Location of Critical Access Hospitals
Information Gathered Through December 17, 2007

Alaska and Hawai not to scale

Legend
( )–N
Critical Access Hospital (1,292)
☐ Metropolitan country
☐ Nonmetropolitan country
■ State not eligible or not participating
Note: Core Based Statistical Areas are current as of the December 2006 update.
Nonmetropolitan countries include micropolitan and countries outside of CBSAs.
Produced by: North Carolina Rural Health Research and Policy Analysis Center, ?? G.
Sheps Center for Health Services Research, University of North Carolina at Chapel Hill.

Sources: US Census Bureau, 2006; CMS Regional Office, ORHP, and State Offices Coordinating with MRHFP, 2007.

Figure 4.3   Location of critical access hospitals: 2007. Source: Rural Assistance Center. "CAH Frequently Asked Questions." September 2008. http://www.raconline.org/ "As of December 2007, there are 1,292 certified Critical Access Hospitals located throughout the United States. The Flex Monitoring Team maintains a list of Critical Access Hospitals which includes the hospital name, city, state, zip code and effective date of CAH status." http://www.raconline.org/info_guides/hospitals/cahfaq.php#howmany

4.3 Types of Hospitals

4.3.1 General Acute Care Hospitals

Also known as medical surgical hospitals or "short stay," these providers offer a range of inpatient services from surgery to pediatrics, obstetrics (labor and delivery), orthopedics, intensive and perhaps cardiac care units, diagnostic services, and outpatient services. General acute care hospitals are defined in part by the kinds of services they perform and by the fact that their patients generally stay for less than 30 days. They may be organized as voluntary nonprofit entities, as private for-profit businesses, or as public organizations owned and managed by a public governing body (federal, state, county, or local government).

4.3.2 Academic Medical Centers and Teaching Hospitals

According to the Association of American Medical Colleges, there are "126 accredited U.S. medical schools that are members of the organization" (4). Of these, approximately 60% are owned by government entities and 40% are owned by private, nonprofit organizations (4). In addition to the 126 allopathic medical schools, there are 25 osteopathic medical schools in the United States.

The organizational structure of *academic medical centers* blossomed in the 1960s when federal legislation and research grants supported the advancement of research and teaching in medical schools. As hospitals and medical schools organized themselves under one governance structure, they provided the infrastructure for research and advanced medical learning. The hospital provided the "laboratory" for research and for clinical exposure to medical practice, and the medical school provided the academic environment for the learning of scientific theory. "Because university medical complexes were increasingly recognized as leading the way toward a more sophisticated and effective healthcare system, the federal government assisted in extending that expertise through the regional medical program legislation of 1965" (5). Under this legislation, research into the leading causes of death was expanded widely: heart disease, cancer, and stroke. University medical complexes, as the centers of research, teaching, and service innovations, gained substantially (5).

Ultimately, many academic medical centers expanded into becoming academic health centers as they added nursing schools, schools of pharmacy, medical technology, and other allied health disciplines. In various organizational arrangements, they either developed their own on-campus allied health school or aligned with local colleges and universities to provide classroom training while the medical center provided clinical practice sites for students.

Teaching hospitals operate in affiliation with medical schools and/or an academic medical center in order to provide specialty training for physicians and other clinicians. In other words, the hospital and the medical school are separate entities (in contrast to the academic medical center in which they are structured under one organizational entity).

The U.S. healthcare system relies heavily on teaching hospitals and their clinics, emergency departments, ambulatory care centers, chronic care facilities, hospices, and individual and group practices for the clinical education of medical students and physician residents. Teaching hospitals serve as "centers for experimental, innovative and technically sophisticated services. Many of the advances started in the research laboratories of medical schools are incorporated into patient care through clinical research programs at teaching hospitals. Additionally, teaching hospitals are special places that help the underserved and provide comprehensive and unique services for the general population" (4).

4.3.3 Specialty Hospitals

Specialty hospitals have been a part of the fabric of U.S. healthcare delivery for the past century. They are hospitals that specialize in performing a limited range of specific medical diagnoses and treatments. Early specialty hospitals were those that served individuals with mental illness and women. Currently, many specialty hospitals are owned by healthcare systems or by physicians, and they specialize in one of several major areas: children or pediatric services, rehabilitation, psychiatric, cancer, cardiology, and orthopedics. There has, in recent years, been an expansion of specialty hospitals by investors, and this phenomenon has been met with resistance by general hospitals and health systems based on concern for the incursion of these specialty hospitals into the markets and high-revenue services, especially cardiac and orthopedic, of existing hospitals and on their concensus that quality of care is lower in certain specialty hospitals. On the other hand, specialty hospital investor owners claim that they can achieve higher quality and greater efficiency by focusing on one service, performing procedures frequently, and gaining expertise through repetition.

4.3.4 Mental Health Hospitals

Mental health hospitals are another classification of hospitals that may be owned by either a governmental or a private entity. They are also known as behavioral health facilities. Historically, it has been the role of state governments to provide needed mental healthcare services within their respective states for persons unable to pay for these services. Consequently, states across the country developed large mental health facilities during the middle of the twentieth century; many of these facilities operated a thousand or more beds and were used more as "warehousing" venues for persons with mental illnesses or other conditions that affected their behavior but that were not diagnosable with the technology of the time.

In the 1970s, the process of "deinstitutionalization" of mental health patients and reintegrating them back into society was launched. "With the development of new psychotropic medications, experts began to believe that patients would be better served outside the mental hospitals" (6). In reality, as state hospitals closed their doors, many of the resident patients of these defunct facilities were left to their own devices or with minimal support from the state. While the federal Mental Health Centers Act of 1963 provided funding for community mental health centers, there were insufficient numbers of them to serve the increasing numbers of people being released from the state hospitals.

Most states continue to operate mental health facilities; however, these are more scaled back in size for inpatient care, and most emphasize outpatient and day treatment. The advances in new drugs to treat mental health conditions have enabled states to effectively address the needs of patients in this less institutionalized setting.

Mental health inpatient facilities are also owned and operated by both nonprofit and for-profit companies. These businesses may specialize in mental health and/or substance abuse treatment and may further specialize in treatment of children and/or young adults. Many of these private companies own facilities and outpatient services across the country or in certain regions, and most, similarly to privately owned acute care hospitals, are not networked for the sharing of patient and financial or operational information.

In all, there are 462 psychiatric facilities in the United States with a total of 84,322 beds. Of these, eight institutions serve individuals with mental retardation, providing 3993 beds. Many hospitals throughout the country also provide psychiatric units. (7)

4.4   Hospital Operations

There are three areas that are essential to gaining an understanding of how hospitals function: (1) the structure of the hospital-physician relationship, (2) the structure of the integrated delivery network (IDN), and (3) how reimbursement for services (i.e., the business model of healthcare) works. The thir area is discussed in chapter 8. In this chapter we focus on the hospital–physician relationship and the structure of the IDN.

4.4.1 The Structure of the Hospital–Physician Relationship

The role of physicians and hospitals has been, for decades, a point of both contention and collaboration for both parties. In understanding healthcare delivery, one key component is to gain an understanding of how physicians and hospitals relate to one another structurally. This structure affects the control they have of their respective businesses, the economic opportunities and challenges that each has, and the ability of each to function and/or to effect change, whether in cost, quality, efficiency, or effectiveness.

Hospitals and doctors have historically functioned as independent but codependent (not meant as a psychological allusion) entities. That is, physicians who admit patients to the hospital and order tests or procedures in the hospital are not salaried employees of the hospital. Their income arises from seeing patients in their offices, from admitting and visiting them in the hospital, and from procedures they do in the hospital or in other settings. The hospital, on the other hand, is totally dependent on physicians to admit patients, to order tests, and to perform procedures on its premises — in other words, the only way the hospital earns income is through the pen stroke (ordering of tests and procedures) of doctors. The hospital, unlike other businesses, can only bill for its clinical services or functions upon a physician's signed order. The hospital carries out that order and can then bill for the service performed. Yet the hospital maintains facilities, technologies, and clinical and administrative staff for each of its services. Similarly to the economic relationship between hospitals and doctors, the hospital's clinical staff (nurses, therapists, laboratory and x-ray technologists, pharmacists, etc.) cannot perform a diagnostic or therapeutic service without the written order of the physician. Consequently, physicians hold not only an economic "ace" over the hospital but also a certain level of authority over the work of the hospital's staff in performing clinical services.

This fundamental economic relationship between doctors and hospitals has been a cause of angst and a driver of collaboration between the two entities for decades: *angst* because each has power over the other (the doctor needs the hospital in order to practice medicine, and the hospital needs the doctor to use its technology and services and cannot earn patient services revenue without the doctor), and *collaboration* because each needs the other in order to function.

The relationship between hospitals and physicians occurs through the mechanism of the medical staff. The medical staff is an organization that gets its authority from the board of the hospital. The board creates and empowers a formally structured organization composed solely of and for physicians and maintains a role in the functioning of the medical staff through bylaws and a committee structure, typically a "joint conference committee," and other committees with specific areas of responsibility (e.g., credentials committee, utilization review committee, infection control committee). The medical staff functions in the pattern of hierarchical organizations with a chief of staff (in other organizations, this would be the equivalent of the CEO — although the chief of staff is a practicing physician in the case of the medical staff), an executive committee, and chairs of various specialties or departments of the hospital (e.g., surgery, orthopedics, pediatrics, gastroenterology). On a day-to-day basis, the chief of staff interacts closely with the president and CEO of the hospital, and it is these two who must forge a working relationship. Each has power over the other's potential for success.

Physicians then gain access to use of the facilities of the hospital for patient admissions, tests, and surgical and other procedures by gaining and holding membership on the medical staff. The physician applies to the medical staff for membership, and the medical staff follows a credentialing process that has been developed by it and approved by the hospital's board of directors. The application for membership is initially reviewed and approved by the credentials committee and is then submitted to the executive committee of the medical staff for approval. With that approval, finalized by the hospital board, the physician is authorized to admit patients, order tests, and treat or perform procedures on patients within the limits of the credentials he or she holds. In other words, the orthopedist, for example, is authorized to use hospital facilities and services for his or her patients only within the range of approval given for his or her specialty.

The process for gaining and retaining credentials is one in which the medical staff looks at all aspects of the physician's credentials and history. It is required to review not only academic and practice credentials but also any history of malpractice or actions taken by other providers or the legal system against the applicant physician.

Membership on the medical staff of a hospital gains the physician access to use of the facilities and services of the hospital in the care of the patient. Outside of medical staff membership, the physician will typically maintain his or her own private practice. That may be a solo practice in which the physician does not have other doctors in the practice or, more typically, a single-specialty practice in which the physician joins with other physicians in the like specialty (e.g., orthopedics, ophthalmology, pediatrics) or a multispecialty practice in which physicians of various specialties work together, share office practices, and refer patients to one another.

While the hospital-physician relationship has been built on a structural model that has inherent tensions, the old model of the medical staff structure is changing. As William Petasnick says in writing for *Frontiers of Health Services Management*: "The old model…governed by the rules of the organized medical staff structure, doesn't work in the current environment, which has grown increasingly complex as a result of legal, economic, and care delivery changes. These complexities make relationship management challenging. Hospitals and physicians struggle to align behavior to achieve cost and quality goals. The need has never been greater for hospitals and physicians to work together as a joint clinical enterprise to improve quality, reduce practice variation, and control the cost of healthcare" (8). In an expanding relationship, hospitals are increasingly hiring primary care physicians or purchasing their practices, and they are hiring physicians to work full-time in the hospital as hospitalists.

4.5   Integrated Delivery Networks

IDNs developed quickly in the 1990s with the proliferation of managed care. As managed care payers structured their business model around achieving negotiated discount rates from healthcare providers, they also implemented a mechanism in which a case manager worked with the provider to ensure that services were used efficiently and not to excess, to achieve acceptable rates of quality and cost reductions. As managed care companies approached the hospital with large numbers of enrolled members (employees and families of major companies), to seek volume discounts from a limited panel of providers, hospitals, physicians, and others recognized quickly the value of size at the negotiating table. They also recognized the value of geographic presence in order to protect their markets and to provide the continuum of care that managed care companies wanted for their enrollees. Larger hospitals began to aggressively pursue acquisition of physician practices, ambulatory care and surgical centers, and other providers who would give them both presence in and access to primary and secondary markets of patients and the continuum of care in which all patient needs would be met within the single organizational entity. In some cases, where acquisition or merger was not possible, affiliations were created to achieve similar purposes. Many continue to expand as they seek size and resources to secure and dominate their markets.

While IDNs create their structures in order to provide a continuum of care for the patient, most of them have not completed the development of the information technology that is fundamental to full integration. Without the information infrastructure to support complete sharing of information between and among all the entities in the IDN, costs are duplicated, tests are duplicated, information is duplicated, and often one provider of care does not know what another has prescribed or tested for any given patient. The current investment of billions of dollars in information technology holds the promise of enabling this kind of sharing and improved decision making when the clinician comes face to face with the patient in whatever venue of care they find themselves.

4.6 Summary

In this chapter, we discussed the major organizational structures under which healthcare providers organize themselves. Whether they are for-profits or not-for-profits and tax-exempt or taxed, each is a vital part of its community. Their efforts to integrate multiple hospitals, nursing care facilities, rehabilitation, ambulatory care, physician practices, and other providers into one organizational entity are ongoing. In the current financial and reimbursement system, the individual provider is hard pressed to "stand alone," whether that is a physician practice, a small hospital, or a surgery center. Each is reliant on a system of referrals and on the sharing of administrative services and of high-priced technology. In the current situation in which there are looming shortages of primary care doctors and nurses, cost cutting, and increasing disparities in access to care, the more providers can do to operate effectively and efficiently and to reduce medical errors, the better chance they have of surviving and thriving.

References

1. HFMA. Fact Sheet: Attributes of Tax Exempt Healthcare Organizations. Accessed November 7, 2007. Available at: http://www.hfma.org/library/compliance/taxexempt/400511+attributes.htm?print=on
2. J. Carlson, 2008. "Unlocking the community chest." *Modern Healthcare*, 16.
3. B. Japsen, 2007. "Hospital Taxes Would Give County $240 Million in Revenue." Chicago Tribune
4. Association of American Medical Colleges (AAMC), 2008. Teaching Hospitals. Accessed December 2008. Available at: http://www.aamc.org/teachinghospitals.htm
5. H. A. Sultz and K. M. Young, 2009. *Health Care USA: Understanding Its Organization and Delivery*, 6th Edition. Jones and Bartlett, Sudbury, MA, p. 159
6. C. Larson, 1998. "Set free: Once considered humane, the wholesale release of mentally ill patients is now under scrutiny." *AHA News*, 9
7. Health Forum, American Hospital Association, 2008. *AHA Hospital Statistics. 2008 Edition*. Health Forum, LLC, Chicago.
8. W. D. Petnasick, 2007. "Hospital-physician relationships: Imperative for clinical enterprise collaboration." *Frontiers of Health Services Management*, 24(1), 3.

Websites

Association of American Medical Colleges (AAMC): http://www.aamc.org

Chapter 5

Doctors in the Healthcare Delivery Structure

5.1   Introduction

When studying the organization of healthcare delivery in the United States, it is important to understand the role of physicians and how that role plays out in the structure of delivery of care. Historically, and still today, physicians and hospitals have a special relationship. As discussed in chapter 4, they are completely interdependent, yet they work under different business models. The way in which physicians are integrated into healthcare delivery is changing as they take on new and expanding roles. While for more than half a century physicians have worked almost exclusively in their own private practices, holding medical staff privileges at local hospitals for admissions, they currently are found in increasing numbers in management roles and on hospital payrolls working as hospitalists, as intensivists, and in other clinical areas. There are approximately 700,000 active doctors in clinical management, research and other roles in the United States.

5.2   Physician Workforce

Of more than 900,000 physicians in the United States, no more than 630,000 were actively practicing medicine in 2006. According to 2005 data from the

American Medical Association as reported by the Bureau of Labor Statistics, only more than 40% of physicians were in the primary care specialties of general internal medicine, family medicine, pediatrics, and obstetrics/gynecology. The balance of almost 60% of physicians practiced in other specialties (see Table 5.1). The United States currently faces a severe shortage of primary care physicians to serve the needs of an aging baby boomer population and the increasing demand for primary care as driven by payers and consumers. However, the median income for primary care physicians is significantly lower than that for certain other specialties, creating a disincentive for medical students to choose a primary care field (Table 5.2). According to

Table 5.1 Selected Physician Specialties in the United States: 1975–2005

	2005		2000		1990	
Specialty						
Internal Medicine	154,002	17.1%	134,539	16.5%	98,349	16.0%
Family medicine	81,701	9.7	71,635	8.8	47,639	7.7
Pediatrics	72,288	8.0	62,386	7.7	40,893	6.6
Obstetrics/ Gynecology	42,600	4.7	40,241	4.9	33,697	5.5
Psychiatry	41,598	4.6	39,457	4.8	35,163	5.7
Anesthesiology	40,494	4.5	35,715	4.4	25,981	4.2
Emergency Medicine*	29,144	3.2	23,064	2.8	14,243	2.3
Diagnostic Radiology	24,231	2.7	21,104	2.6	15,412	2.5
Orthopedic Surgery	24,140	2.7	22,287	2.7	19,138	3.1
Cardiovascular Dis.	22,349	2.5	21,025	2.6	15,862	2.6
Other	369,506	41.0	342,317	42.1	269,044	43.7

Data were not available for Emergency Medicine prior to 1980.

Source: American Medical Association. "Physician Characteristics and Distribution in the U.S." American Medical Association Press, 2007.

the *Journal of the American Medical Association*, the United States may have a shortage of as many as 85,000 physicians by 2020.

Before we delve into this further, let us start at the beginning and consider how doctors are trained in the United States.

5.3 How Are Doctors Trained?

Medical schools are organized within one of two overall medical disciplines: allopathy and osteopathy. Allopathy is defined as "a philosophy of medicine that views medical treatment as active intervention to counteract the effects of disease through medical and surgical procedures that produce effects opposite to those of the disease" (1, 581) or as a "therapeutic system in which a disease is treated by producing a second condition that is incompatible with or antagonistic to the first" (2). Osteopathy on the other hand "is a medical philosophy based on the holistic approach to treatment. It uses the traditional methods of medical practice, which includes pharmaceuticals, laboratory tests, X-ray diagnostics, and surgery, and supplements them by advocating treatment that involves correction of the position of the joints or tissues and by emphasizing diet and environment as factors that might destroy natural resistance" (pp. 591–592) (1). It is important to understand that even though allopathic and osteopathic physicians are trained in

Table 5.2 Median Compensation for Physicians in Selected Specialties: 2005

Specialty	Less than Two Years in Specialty	Over One Year in Specialty
Anesthesiology	$259,948	$321,686
Surgery: General	228,839	282,504
Obstetrics/gynecology: General	203,270	247,348
Psychiatry: General	173,922	180,000
Internal medicine: General	141,912	166,420
Pediatrics: General	132,953	161,331
Family practice (without obstetrics)	137,119	156,010

Source: Bureau of Labor Statistics – Occupational Outlook Handbook, 2008–2009 Edition. Accessed December 2008. Available at: http://www.bls.gov/oco/ocos074.htm

different philosophical approaches to disease and healing, both complete similar rigorous didactic and clinical training and both are required to pass a licensure examination in order to practice medicine in the United States.

5.3.1 Number of Medical Schools and Their Enrollments

Today there are 129 medical school programs (allopathic) and another 25 osteopathic medical college programs leading to the M.D. degree in the United States. Enrollment in these programs was at a total of just more than 66,000 medical students each year until 2004, when those numbers started to increase. In 2007, there were slightly more than 70,000 students in medical schools in the United States (Table 5.3). The proportion of male to female medical students changed significantly from 1992 to 2007 to a point at which there were almost as many women actively enrolled in medical school as there were men (Figure 5.1 and Table 5.4). In 2007, there were about 36,000 male medical students and 34,000 female students enrolled (3).

Of the 70,000 medical students, 16,139 graduated in 2007. As Figure 5.2 demonstrates, the number of graduates increased only slightly since 2002, when they totaled 15,676. This is an increase of less than 3%. The gender profile of graduates mirrors that of enrollees (3) (Figure 5.2).

5.3.2 Typical Course of Study in Medical School

Having gotten a sense of the number of physicians trained in the United States, a review of the course of training that they complete will help deepen the understanding of both the scope and the content of their work.

The typical medical school curriculum is broken down into two parts and designed around the progression of the student through the education program. Entering students are required to have a premedical education grounded in the sciences. In the first and second years of medical school, students primarily work in the classroom learning basic sciences; the third and fourth years are spent primarily out of the classroom and in the clinical setting gaining experience in working with inpatients and with outpatients in teaching hospitals or academic medical centers.

Table 5.3 Physician Characteristics and Distribution in the United States: 1970–2005

	2005		2000		1990		1980		1970	
Gender										
Male	657,140	73%	618,233	76%	511,227	83.1%	413,395	88.4%	308,627	92.4%
Female	244,913	27	195,537	24	104,194	16.9	54,284	11.6	25,401	7.6
Total	902,053		813,869		615,421		467,679		334,028	
Age										
Under 35	140,093	16%	136,704	17%	134,872	22%	275,506	45%	88,413	26%
35–64	592,115	66	533,127	65	385,160	63	275,142	45	208,270	62
65 and over	169,845	19	144,939	18	95,389	15	64,031	10	41,321	12
Professional Activity									1975*	
Office-based patient care	563,225	62.4%	490,398	60.3%	360,995	58.7%	272,000	58.2%	215,429	54.7%
Hospital based patient care	155,248	17.2	157,032	19.3	142,875	23.2	104,512	22.3	96,508	24.5
Residents/Fellows**	95,391	10.6	95,725	11.8	92,080	15.0	62,042	13.3	57,802	14.7
Full-Time Staff	59,857	6.6	61,307	7.5	50,795	8.3	42,470	9.1	38,706	9.8
Other professional activity***	43,965	4.9	44,938	5.5	43,440	7.1	38,404	8.2	28,343	7.2
Inactive	99,823	11.1	75,168	9.2	52,653	8.6	25,744	5.5	21,449	5.4
Not Classified	39,304	4.4	45,136	5.5	12,678	2.1	20,629	4.4	26,145	6.6
Address Unknown	488	0.1	1,098	0.1	2,780	0.5	6,390	1.4	5,868	1.5

* 1975 data presented for professional activity.

** Includes all years of residency.

*** Includes Administration, medical teaching, research activities, research fellows, and other.

Source: American Medical Association. "Physician Characteristics and Distribution in the U.S." American Medical Association Press, 2007.

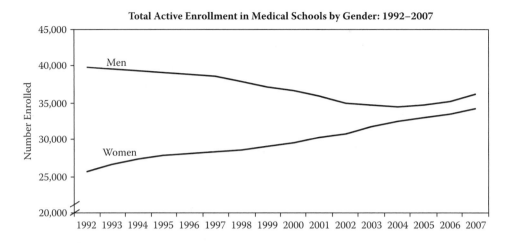

Figure 5.1   Total active enrollment in U.S. medical schools by sex: 1992–2007. Sources: Association of American Medical Colleges. *AAMC Data Warehouse: Student section as of January 16, 2002.* Total enrollment is reported as of October 31 of the academic year. Association of American Medical Colleges. *AAMC: Data Warehouse: STUDENT File, as of 12/6/2007.* (http://www.aamc.org/data/facts/start.htm)

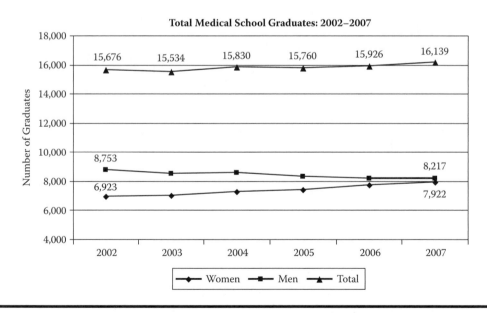

Figure 5.2   Total U.S. medical school graduates: 2002–2007. Source: AAMC: Data Warehouse: Student file, as of 9/19/2007 (http://www.aamc.org/data/facts/2007/schoolgrads0207.htm)

5.3.3 Preclinical Curriculum/Basic Sciences

Although students have clinical experiences throughout medical school, the first two years are often called the "preclinical" phase of their education. The preclinical phase typically occupies the first 2 years after entering school. The basic science departments are largely responsible for the content of the preclinical curriculum, where the normal structure and function of human systems are taught through gross and microscopic anatomy, biochemistry, physiology, behavioral science, and neuroscience. After students' completion of the basic sciences, the educational focus shifts to abnormalities of the body's structure and function, disease, and general therapeutic principles through courses in microbiology, immunology, pharmacology, and pathology.

After the second year of medical school, students take the first of a series of national exams, the United States Medical Licensing Examination or USMLE. Passing this examination is key to continuing on in medical school.

5.3.4 Clinical Phase

Having successfully completed step 1 of the USMLE, the student moves into the third or junior year of medical school. The clinical phase of the curriculum usually occurs during the last 2 years of medical school and is devoted to education in the clinical setting. These periods of instruction are called clerkships, and they may range in length from approximately 4 to 12 weeks. During clerkships, students work with patients and their families in inpatient and outpatient settings.

Required "core" clerkships in all schools include internal medicine, pediatrics, psychiatry, surgery, obstetrics/gynecology, and family medicine. Depending on the school, required clerkships can also include other specialties such as family medicine, primary care, neurology, and community or rural medicine.

While in a hospital setting or a hospital clinic, students work under the supervision of physician faculty members (known as "attending physicians") and physician residents, and they work with other members of the healthcare team, including nurses, social workers, psychologists, pharmacists, and other technical staff. Students frequently experience "preceptorships" — that is, they are assigned to community physicians' offices to gain first-hand knowledge about how a practice of medicine functions (4).

After this fourth year, the student completes the second part of the national boards or USMLE (5).

5.3.5 Licensing

Upon successful completion of the USMLE, the graduate then goes on to complete the licensing examination of the respective state in which he or she plans to practice. Individual states are responsible for the licensing of physicians, and in doing so their requirements will vary depending on state legislation and on the unique requirements of the state. Upon successful completion of the state licensing examination, the newly minted physician can go on to practice general medicine. However, the more typical progression is for the physician to enter a medical residency in a specialty in which he or she intends to practice (e.g., orthopedics, otolaryngology, pediatrics, surgery).

5.3.6 Graduate Medical Education: Becoming a Specialist

Residencies are offered at teaching hospitals and academic medical centers. Their physician faculty combine both an active, albeit part-time, medical office practice in a "faculty practice plan" and devote time to supervising the training of residents within the specific specialties for which they and the hospital or medical center are approved. Residencies for medical specialization last from 3 to 5 years, depending on the specialty chosen; if the physician then decides to pursue a sub-specialty (e.g., retinal specialist is a sub-specialty of ophthalmology), he or she will spend another 1 to 3 years completing a *fellowship* in the sub-specialty.

Upon completion of the specialty residency, physicians must successfully complete an examination given by their respective specialty board for the area in which they will practice. The American Board of Medical Specialties is the overarching body of which 24 specialty boards are members. Together, they offer 145 specialty and sub-specialty certifications (6).

Finally, having completed a specialty and/or sub-specialty, board-certified physicians are required to maintain that certification through the Maintenance of Certification of the American Board of Medical Specialties. The Maintenance of Certification requires ongoing medical education so that the physician can maintain skills and stay abreast of advances in the field and assessments or examinations in which the specialist must demonstrate continuing skill in the specialty that are given periodically. The requirements for continuing medical education may vary by state.

Table 5.4 Medical School Enrollment in the United States

	Men	*Women*	*Total*
1992	39,830	25,745	65,575
1993	39,593	26,582	66,175
1994	39,429	27,359	66,788
1995	39,016	27,926	66,942
1996	38,761	28,165	66,926
1997	38,497	28,399	66,896
1998	37,897	28,642	66,539
1999	37,253	29,124	66,377
2000	36,625	29,535	66,160
2001	35,972	30,281	66,253
2002	35,042	30,792	65,834
2003	34,585	31,715	66,300
2004	34,414	32,610	67,024
2005	34,678	33,037	67,715
2006	35,220	33,533	68,753
2007	36,126	34,099	70,225

Sources: Association of American Medical Colleges. AAMC Data Warehouse: Student section as of January 16, 2002. Total enrollment is reported as of October 31 of the academic year. Association of American Medical Colleges. AAMC: Data Warehouse: Student file, as of 12/6/2007. (http://www.aamc. org/data/facts/start.htm)

5.4   International Medical Graduates

The United States admits about 6,000 international medical graduates (IMGs) to residencies and fellowships each year. Of these, about 1150 are U.S. IMGs (i.e., U.S. citizens who started medical school in other countries) and about 4800 are non-U.S. IMGs (i.e., medical school graduates who are not U.S. citizens but who are certified to enter a residency or fellowship in the United States) (see Table 5.5). Educational Commission for Foreign Medical Graduates (ECFMG) certification is required of all IMGs to enter a residency or fellowship in the United States.

IMGs entering residencies in the United States tend to enter what are considered primary care specialties — general internal medicine, pediatrics,

Table 5.5 Certified International Medical Graduates (IMGs) Entering Residency Programs: 1995–2003

Entry Year	Total	U.S. IMGs		Non-U.S. IMGs	
		Number	Percent	Number	Percent
1995	5,410	413	7.6	4,997	92.4
1996	5,379	514	9.6	4,865	90.4
1997	5,414	674	12.5	4,740	87.5
1998	5,371	908	16.9	4,463	83.1
1999	5,905	1,049	17.8	4,856	82.2
2000	6,907	1,415	23.2	4,682	76.8
2001	6,170	1,453	23.6	4,717	76.5
2002	6,208	1,373	22.1	4,835	77.9
2003	6,004	1,150	19.2	4,854	80.8

Source: Retrieved December 4, 2008, from, American Medical Association. Educational Commission for Foreign Medical Graduates, 2007 Presentation. Website: www. ama-assn.org

family medicine, and obstetrics/gynecology. As indicated in Table 5.6, about 36% of all physicians in internal medicine in the United States are IMGs, 28% of pediatritians are IMGs, and just less than 18% of family medicine physicians are IMGs.

Table 5.6 Primary Specialty of International Medical Graduates (IMGs)

Specialty	Number of IMG Physicians	Percentage in Specialty (%)
Internal Medicine	55,467	36
Psychiatry	13,080	31.4
Anesthesiology	11,757	29
Pediatrics	20,180	28
General Surgery	7,597	20
Radiology	1,653	18.8
Family Medicine	21,669	17.8
Obstetrics/Gynecology	7,589	17.8

Source: American Medical Association. Physician Characteristics and Distribution in the U.S. Chicago: American Medical Association, 2007.

5.5 Financial Support of Medical Education

Historically, medical schools have relied on a number of revenue sources. The clinical practice of faculty has been a significant source of funding — up to one-third of total medical school income is generated by the faculty from the patient care they deliver in the Faculty Practice Plan (i.e., a "group practice" in which they have scheduled office hours to see patients). Research grants and contracts provide just less than 20% of funding needs, and a portion of support is also derived from endowments. Much of the balance of funding has come from Medicare and Medicaid's subsidization of graduate medical education (GME). However, that support has been gradually diminishing, and this scaling back of subsidies for GME has reduced revenues for academic medical centers and teaching hospitals. Additionally, "available data suggest that hospitals affiliated with academic health centers are 20% to 30% more expensive than other hospitals" (7) — a reality that reflects the cost of medical education and the availability of state-of-the-art technologies in medical training specialties. In this era of increasing financial pressure on hospitals, there is strong pressure on teaching hospitals and medical schools to find other means of support for medical education.

5.6 How Doctors Work with Hospitals

As discussed in chapter 4, doctors are credentialed by and admitted to membership on the medical staff of a hospital prior to being permitted to perform procedures or admit patients to the hospital. The hospital does not pay salaries to most of its admitting doctors; instead, the role of the hospital is to provide the technology, staff, structures, and processes that support the physician in his or her medical practice related to inpatients' and outpatients' diagnostic and therapeutic services. In chapter 4, we discussed this process through which physicians gain access to admit and treat their patients in hospitals. The medical staff, which is a formally organized body under the authority of the hospital's board of directors, is the physicians' organizational structure in the hospital. In working with healthcare providers, it is very important to understand this organizational structure and its impact on the way in which the hospital operates. It is key to the business model of both the doctor and the hospital.

There are certain specialties whose role is structured differently in the hospital. In addition to the role of the private practice physician on the medical staff of the hospital, certain specialist physicians work within the hospital under contract to provide core services. These contract physicians include radiologists, pathologists, emergency department doctors, and anesthesiologists.

Except for emergency department physicians, contract physicians do not admit patients, but their service is an essential part of the hospital process. These physicians may be the medical heads or directors of their respective departments, and they staff and provide specialized services to support the diagnosis and treatment of patients. They do not receive a salary from the hospital but bill for their portion of each test (e.g., reading an X-ray) or treatment that they provide.

In yet another structural model, certain physicians also work as employees of hospitals and health systems. Their roles include employed primary care physicians in office practice; hospitalists and intensivists; and physicians in upper management of the hospital (CEOs, medical directors, CMOs, CMIOs, etc.).

The number of employed primary care physicians is growing as hospitals expand their networks to provide essential services in selected markets, to manage the quality and costs of care, and to stabilize the scope of their services. For physicians, the lower salary they might receive as an employee of the hospital is a welcome tradeoff from having to work long office hours in private practice. They are happy to gain an improved work–life balance and to be removed from the demands of managing an office, the complexities of health insurance systems, decreasing revenue pressures from government and private payers, and increasing costs of doing business (including malpractice insurance).

The traditional role of physicians in hospitals and that of the medical staff structure are under ongoing review and change to meet the needs of a changing healthcare system. Physicians are increasingly moving into newly defined roles in the hospital. The role of hospitalists and intensivists is a recent development in healthcare. Hospitals have engaged in hiring physicians to provide in-hospital medical care to patients who are admitted to the hospitals. These physicians, however, do not admit patients to the hospital. Hospitalists work in the inpatient units of the hospital, and intensivists work specifically in the intensive care and cardiac care units. In both instances, when a patient's doctor admits him or her, that patient's in-hospital care is provided by the hospitalist. Except for many specialities, the admitting doctor does not need to visit the patient or manage his or her care while admitted to the hospital. This works particularly well for primary care physicians and certain specialists who would otherwise be required to share 24/7 coverage of their hospitalized inpatients (i.e., be on call at scheduled hours of the day, night, and weekends). Hospitalists and intensivists are paid a salary by the hospital and are scheduled to work regular staff hours.

Physicians in *management roles* are also increasing in hospitals. They may be the president/CEO of the hospital, the chief medical officer, or chief medical information officer, or may serve as chief of overall clinical services or in any other similar position of authority. In these roles, the physician spends little to no time in the direct care of patients and instead is responsible for the management of resources, for interrelationships, and for other strategic and administrative duties.

5.7   The Physician's Source(s) of Income

A key factor regarding the doctor's work in the hospital is that most doctors who admit patients to the hospital and perform surgery or other procedures are not employees of the hospital — the hospital does not pay them a salary. While some doctors are hired by the hospital to work as hospitalists or intensivists and others are hired to work in the management of the hospital, most admitting physicians are not employed or paid by the hospital. Neither does the hospital bill the insurance company on behalf of the doctor. That leaves the doctor to do his or her own billing for services.

The doctor's primary income is from his or her clinical care of patients. In addition, he or she may earn income from other investments, educational and speaking engagements, and there may be other non-clinical sources of income that the doctor might have. Physicians bill directly for the patient visits, diagnosis, and treatments that they perform in their private offices. In doing this, they are required to comply with all the rules of the many private and government payers who provide health insurance. Most insurance payers enter into contractual arrangements with doctors in which the fee for each service the doctor provides is negotiated and discounted to what the insurer is willing to pay for the respective service. In each case, the doctor agrees to the amount that is to be paid and concurrently agrees not to "balance bill" the patient. In other words, if the doctor's established fee for an office visit is $95 and the payer agrees to pay $45, then the doctor can only collect the co-pay from the patient (e.g., $15) and cannot bill that patient for the balance, which in our example would be $35. The level of discount varies by payer and may vary yet more in Medicare and Medicaid billings, which are also deeply discounted reimbursement programs.

The concept of balance billing becomes more complicated when the patient makes a visit to a physician or hospital that is not in the network of providers approved by his or her insurance payer. In this case, the provider is not bound by a payment agreement with the insurer. While that insurer may pay the portion of the fee that is equal or near the amount that would be paid to an in-network provider, the balance between the full charge and the discounted payment is frequently charged to the patient. While some states may consider this to be illegal or questionable, in many areas such balance billing often takes the patient by surprise.

We have described one source from which the physician receives income for clinical practice. The physician also bills insurers for clinical visits to patients in hospitals and for treatments or procedures performed in hospitals and ambulatory centers. If, for example, a dermatologist performs an out-patient surgical procedure in an ambulatory center, then that dermatologist directly bills the patient's insurer or health plan for the physician's role in that procedure.

5.8 Malpractice

While chapter 7 addresses some of the public policy actions that have been taken to address the crisis in malpractice that the United States has faced, it is appropriate to discuss the topic briefly here in this overview of physicians and their profession in the United States. Malpractice has frequently been the subject of heated and intense discussion. This comes from two perspectives. On the one hand, many physicians pay very high premiums (some say disproportionately high) for their malpractice insurance, particularly in certain specialties such as obstetrics/gynecology. On the other hand, patients who are injured in a medical error or through negligence often feel that they deserve to be financially "made whole" and/or to be assured that the same error is not repeated. They may turn to litigation in this situation. According to the 2001 article "When Doctors Get Sued," about 50%–65% of practicing physicians are sued at least once during their careers (8).

The National Practitioner Data Bank (NPDB) reported that 191,804 medical malpractice lawsuits were reported during the period 1990–2004 (10). Just a few interesting statistics regarding medical malpractice: the Bureau of Justice statistics indicate that in 75 of the largest counties in the United States, medical malpractice plaintiffs won 27% of the cases in 2001. In the following year, overall, 18,999 medical malpractice payment reports were made (9).

The NPDB was created by the U.S. Congress as one initiative to address the growing crisis in medical malpractice litigation and to improve quality of care in the United States. The NPDB receives reports of malpractice payments and adverse actions concerning healthcare practitioners. Adverse actions are those taken against physicians subsequent to a finding of error or wrongdoing on their part. The adverse actions may be related to their licensure, clinical privileges, professional society membership, and participation in Medicare and Medicaid. When adverse actions are taken, that information is reported to the NPDB and then made available to approved entities for review when considering an action relative to an individual physician, such as the granting of medical staff privileges to admit and treat patients in a hospital. It is essentially an alert or flagging system meant to support comprehensive reviews of physicians. It is however confidential, and only authorized entities can gain access to it. It is not available to the public.

5.9   Physician Supply

By 2020, the United States is expected to need between 1.093 and 1.17 million physicians. In similar forecasts, the supply of physicians is expected to be only 1.02 million. The increasing demand for physicians is driven in part by the aging of the baby boom population, which is expected to expand the ranks of persons aged 65 years and older from 35 million in 2004 to 54 million in 2020. Consequently, the country may face a shortage of 70,000 or more physicians in 2020. A combination of factors is converging to drive this shortage (see Table 5.7), including the number of physicians who are changing their lifestyles by working fewer hours, larger numbers of them working in non-patient care settings (e.g., in management and information technology), possible decreases in the number of IMGs entering the country, and changing reimbursement levels. On the consumer side of the equation, we are living longer and will demand more physician services, medical advances offer new options to address disease and disability, and genetic testing is opening new doors to cures and personalized medicine. Exacerbating the looming shortage is the difficulty of increasing the supply of physicians. Medical education is, at a minimum, an 8- to 10-year enterprise for medical training programs. Prior to being able to expand medical education medical school capacity must be expanded and there needs to be sufficient supply of physician faculty to teach. In other words, in highly skilled professions such as medicine, the solution to undersupply is typically a long-range and expensive proposition — both cost and time are the arbiters of a solution to a projected serious lack of physicians in the next decade.

Table 5.7 Physician Supply, Demand, Need, and Factors for Shortage

Supply

- Supply is expected to rise from 781,200 FTEs in 200 to 971,800 in 2020 — a 24% increase.
- The per capita numbers of physicians (per 100,000 persons) are forecast at 283 in 2000, 301 in 2015, and 298 in 2020.
- The most probable aggregate of supply of physicians is 1.02 million FTEs in 2020.

Demand

- Demand will grow to between 1.03 and 1.24 million physicians in 2020.
- Projected U.S. populated growth is 50 million (18% between 2000 and 2020).
- The aging of the population (over 65 years old) will increase from 35 million in 2000. to 54 million in 2020.
- The age-specific per capita physician utilization rates are changing with those under 45 using fewer services and those over 45 using more services.

Need

- Need is projected to grow between 1.09 and 1.17 million physicians in 2020.
- The nation is projected to face a shortage of physicians of between 85,00 and 96,000 in 2020.

Factors Affecting Shortage

- There is a changing lifestyle of working fewer hours.
- Rate of increase in the use of physicians over age 45 will continue.
- Expected increase in the nation's wealth will result in more demand.
- There is a potential increase in non-patient care activities.
- There is a potential reduction in number of hours worked by physicians over 50 and residents.
- Possible decrease in IMG immigration.
- There is a decreasing number of patients, called boutique medicine.
- Advances in genetic testing result in use of more services.
- Medical advances keep individuals alive longer without curing the illness.

Source: U.S. Department of Health and Human Services, Health Resources and Services Administration, Council on Graduate Medical Education, 2005. "Council on Graduate Medical Education Sixteenth Report: Physician Workforce Policy Guidelines for the United States, 2000–2020." Available at: http://www.cogme.gov/16.pdf

5.10 Summary

The role of physicians in healthcare is complex. Functioning as independent practitioners, they are integrally tied to hospitals and healthcare systems. The mutual interdependency of hospitals and doctors has long been a source of angst and has resulted in continually evolving roles and adaptation. For anyone wanting to work effectively among hospitals and doctors, an understanding of this relationship, its challenges, and its impact on the delivery of medical care is essential. Looking to the future, the United States is facing a substantial shortage of physicians, particularly physicians in primary care specialties. This need will drive us to both expand medical education and to find new sources of providing primary care (e.g., through nurse practitioners and physician assistants). In all, the way in which this expansion is financed will determine if we will be able to meet the needs of a growing population.

References

1. L. Shi and D. A. Singh, 2001. *Delivering Health Care in America: A Systems Approach.* Aspen Publishers: Gaithersburg, MD, p. 581
2. American Association of Colleges of Osteopathic Medicine, 2006. "Educational Council on Osteopathic Principles (ECOP) of the Glossary of Osteopathic Terminology Usage Guide." Accessed October 2008. Available at: http://www.osteopathic.org
3. Association of American Medical Colleges, 2007. "AAMC Data Warehouse: Student Section as of January 16, 2002." Accessed October 2008. Available at: http://www.aamc.org/data/facts/start.htm
4. Association of American Medical Colleges, 2008. "Curriculum Directory." Accessed October 2008. Available at: http://services.aamc.org/currdir/about.cfm
5. Medical School Admissions, 2007. Accessed October 2008. Available at: http://www.medical-school.ws/
6. American Board of Medical Specialties, 2008. "Who We Are & What We Do." Accessed October 2008. Available at: http://www.abms.org/About_ABMS/who_we_are.aspx
7. G. F. Anderson, G. Greenberg, and C. K. Lisk, 1999. "**Academic health centers: Exploring a financial paradox.**" *Health Affairs*, 8(2): 156–167.
8. A. M. Dodge and S. F. Fitzer, 2006. *When Good Doctors Get Sued: A Guide for Physicians Involved in Malpractice Lawsuits.* Dodge & Associates: Olalla, WA.

9. U.S. Department of Health and Human Services, Health Resources and Services Administration, Bureau of Health Professions, Division of Practitioner Data Banks, 2006. "National Practitioner Data Bank, 2006 Annual Report". Available at: http://www.npdb-hipdb.hrsa.gov/pubs/stats/2006_NPDB_Annual_Report.pdf

Web sites

American Association of Colleges of Osteopathic Medicine (AACOM): http://www.osteopathic.org
American Board of Medical Specialties (ABMS): http://www.abms.org
Association of American Medical Colleges (AAMC): http://www.aamc.org
Medical School Admissions: http://www.medical-school.ws

Chapter 6

Workforce
Nurses and Others

6.1 Introduction

The healthcare provider sector workforce is composed of widely varying arrays of professional clinical specialties, support staff, and administrative personnel. These professionals and staff find positions working not just in hospitals but also in nursing homes, home health agencies, physician offices, clinics, pharmacies, emergency services, hospice programs, ambulatory settings, diagnostic labs, and other settings. Concurrent to the growth of the healthcare provider sector, the demand for trained allied health clinicians (a broad term that includes nurses, laboratory and radiology technologists, pharmacists, therapists, and other licensed clinicians) has grown and continues to grow. Estimates that we subsequently discuss in this chapter suggest that the United States will be significantly lacking in certain licensed clinical professions (e.g., nursing) by the end of the next decade.

6.2 Nursing

Nursing is by far the largest single profession in the hospital or health system's workforce. Nursing may comprise up to 50% of that workforce. Similarly to physicians on the medical staff, nurses are divided among a number of clinical departments in the hospital, and many become specialized in their clinical area of choice — pediatrics, emergency services, surgery, obstetrics, and so on. They also function at various levels of certification of licensure including Advanced Practice Nurses (APN), Registered Nurses (RN), and licensed pratical or licensed vocational nurses (LPN/LVN).

There were approximately 2,468,340 registered nurses (RNs) working in the United States in 2007 (1). Data from the Department of Health and Human Services relative to RN employment from 1980 through 2004 (Figure 6.1) indicate a steady growth in the number of RNs in the workforce. They also indicate that fewer than 500,000 nurses were not in the workforce in 2004.

Figure 6.2 depicts the major sectors of healthcare in which RNs worked in the 2007. Among these, general medical surgical hospitals employ the greatest percentage. Fully 57% of RNs worked in hospitals, 9% worked in physician offices, and 5% worked in home healthcare and nursing care facilities. About 20% of RNs worked in "other" settings. These include research, teaching, vendor companies, consulting, insurance, and similar venues in which they generally do not work directly with patients.

Also, unlike most physicians, nurses in hospitals work as salaried or hourly staff. They report within the hierarchy of the nursing department in the hospital and typically will function in different nursing roles, from that of "unit nurse" in one of the clinical departments to charge nurses in those departments, to nursing managers, and hierarchically up to a director or

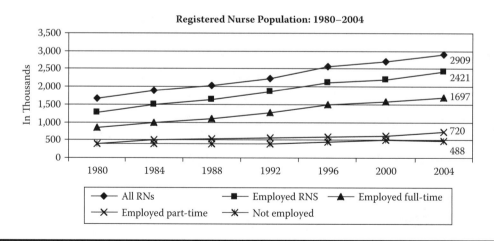

Figure 6.1   Registered nurse population: 1980–2004. Source: U.S. Department of Health and Human Services, Health Resources and Services Administration, Bureau of Health Professionals. "The Registered Nurse Population." March 2004. ftp://ftp.hrsa.gov/bhpr/workforce/0306rnss.pdf

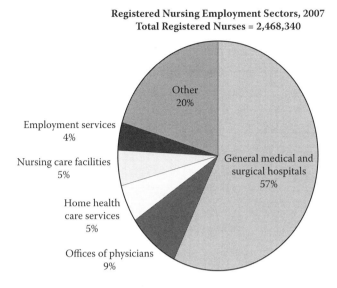

Registered Nursing Employment Sectors, 2007
Total Registered Nurses = 2,468,340

Figure 6.2 Registered nursing employment sectors: 2007. Source: U.S. Department of Labor, Bureau of Labor Statistics. Occupational Employment Statistics — Registered Nurses, 2007. Accessed October 22, 2008. http://www.bls.gov/oes/current/oes291111.htm#ind

vice president of nursing (perhaps of clinical care). Nursing departments are staffed around the clock and work in a "matrix" type of arrangement in which the physicians issue orders for any clinical work that is to be done for patients and in which the nursing management is responsible for ensuring that adequate and qualified nurses are hired, scheduled, and receive continuing education; that budgets are met; that quality mechanisms are in place and followed; and that nursing and patient care goals and objectives are met.

Just as the relationship between physicians and hospital managements has been historically challenging for the reasons discussed in chapter 5, the relationship between nurses and physicians is also often challenging. The physician who is domineering or autocratic may create a perception that the nurse is less than capable. Many nurses have complained of a hostile environment that is disruptive to their functioning as professionals (2). This is one of many reasons why the nursing profession has become unattractive to some who practice it or to others who consider training in the profession. While to many nursing is a very fulfilling and rewarding profession, the instense atmosphere in which they work is only accentuated by what they perceive as pay that is too low, unpredictable or undesirable work hours, long and intense work hours, insufficient staff, and an excess of paperwork (2).

6.2.1 Nursing Shortage

As stated above, in the United States today, there are approximately 2,500,000 registered nurses in the workforce. Figure 6.3 outlines the trend in nursing supply since 2000 and through 2020. It is expected that there will be an undersupply of more than 1 million nurses by 2020. As the U.S. General Accounting Office reported, "[a] serious shortage of nurses is expected in the future as demographic pressures influence both supply and demand" (3). The demand for RNs is expected to increase significantly as baby boomers enter their retirement years. As demographic shifts occur and the number of uninsured increases, access to healthcare may be limited unless the number of nurses and that of other primary caregivers increase in proportion to the increase in demand.

While there is ongoing interest in expanding the number and capacities of nursing schools throughout the United States, this may be only a partial solution to the problem of the growing nursing shortage. Studies of the drivers of the nursing shortage reveal that there are other systemic reasons that also need to be addressed in finding a permanent solution to this particular workforce issue. These drivers include economic issues among nurses who feel there is not sufficient parity of their compensation with others working in clinical services, expanding opportunities for nurses to work in situations in which they are not providing direct care (e.g., in research, sales, quality,

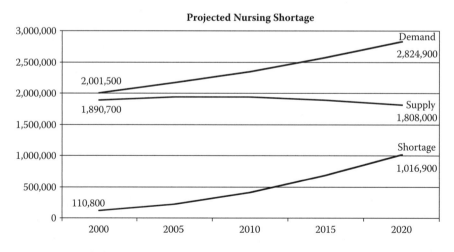

Figure 6.3   Projected nursing shortage. Source: U.S. Department of Labor, Bureau of Labor Statistics. "What is Behind HRSA's Projected Supply, Demand and Shortage of Registered Nurses?" September 2004. Accessed October 22, 2008. Available at: ftp:// ftp.hrsa.gov/bhpr/workforce/behindshortage.pdf

payer, and public policy positions), the often stressful work environment in the clinical setting, insufficient staffing in inpatient units, and the pace and scheduling of work life that requires round-the-clock staffing. Each of these factors will also need to be considered in order to effectively address the serious looming shortage of nurses in the United States.

6.3 Registered Nurses

The role of the RN is played out in a wide variety of settings. The RN is responsible for assessment of patients using their training, experience, and clinical judgment to perform nursing diagnosis, treatment, and evaluation of the progress of the patient and the effectiveness of patient care. The nurse plays a key role in the nursing team that designs the care plan for a patient according to that patient's condition. The clinical settings in which RNs are found include (1)

- ambulatory care
- critical, intensive, and neonatal care
- emergency, trauma, and transport
- home healthcare
- hospice and palliative care
- long-term care
- medical–surgical units of hospitals
- occupational health
- perioperative (preoperative, in the operating room, and in recovery postsurgery)
- physician offices
- psychiatric–mental health services
- radiology
- rehabilitation
- transplant services

6.3.1 Registered Nursing Education

There is a uniquely structured set of alternative educational paths by which an individual can achieve nursing education. According to the American Nurses Association, an individual aspiring to become an RN can acquire a bachelor's degree in nursing (BSN), a diploma in nursing, or an associate degree in nursing (ADN).

- ■ The BSN requires four years of study:
  - – It provides the nursing theory, sciences, humanities, and behavioral science preparation needed for the full scope of professional nursing responsibilities.
  - – It also provides the educational background for advanced education that is required for an advanced practice degree and for specialization in clinical practice and research.
  - – In 2005, 573 U.S. colleges and universities offered the BSN or an advanced nursing degree.
  - – In 2004, 34.2% of all RNs were bachelor's prepared.
- ■ A diploma in nursing requires three years of study:
  - – It combines classroom and clinical instruction.
  - – It has diminished steadily to 4% of all basic RN education programs in 2006 as nursing education has shifted from hospitals to academic institutions.
  - – In 2004, 17.5% of all RNs held a diploma in nursing.
- ■ An ADN requires two years of study:
  - – It prepares individuals for a defined technical scope of practice.
  - – In 2005, associate degree programs were 58.9% of all U.S. basic nursing programs.
  - – In 2004, 33.7% of all RNs held an ADN (4).

6.3.2 RN Licensing

Upon graduation from a state-approved school of nursing, the aspiring RN must pass the NCLEX-RN to obtain a license and to use the RN title. Continuing education or competency requirements are established by state boards of nursing, which also handle disciplinary actions against RNs. Once licensed, the RN must practice in accordance with the requirements of the nurse practice act in the state in which he or she functions. RN licensure is reciprocal among many states, but the RN who wants to practice in another state must apply to that state's board of nursing in order to receive the reciprocal nursing license. This applies to "traveling nurses" who accept temporary assignments in states other than the one in which they hold their original license to practice (4).

6.3.3 Advanced Practice Nurses

Advanced practice nurses (APNs) are those who earn a master's degree in nursing and go on to work as nurse practitioners (NPs), nurse midwives, or nurse anesthetists or clinical nurse specialists. The broader field of nursing offers these clinicians the opportunity to train and work at varying levels of expertise or specialty. Figure 6.4 indicates that more than 50% of APNs work as NPs and that almost 25% are clinical nurse specialists (CNSs). APNs work generally at the bedside or in physician practices and are found in hospitals and in settings such as long-term care and home care. The training that each of these levels requires is outlined in Figure 6.4.

In each of these advanced nursing practices, the professional is required to gain a state license to practice. Nurses who are licensed as NPs have authority to issue a limited range of pharmaceutical prescriptions, work more independently than RNs, and work without the direct supervision or orders of a physician. The range of what they are permitted to do varies by state. They are often described as "physician extenders," particularly in that they may perform certain primary care levels of work as they work in a specialist's office (e.g., taking patient histories, providing patient education, and following up on surgical procedures) or they are authorized to diagnose common conditions and to prescribe drugs and treatments within a limited range in the primary care setting. NPs are authorized to bill directly for their services under many governmental and private payer arrangements.

Nurse midwives are also specially licensed by individual states to assist in obstetrical care and at the delivery of infants. This field of nursing has a long history as it developed out of a need for labor and delivery nurses in rural and underserved areas in the nineteenth and twentieth centuries. Financially, nurse midwives bill payers directly for their services. They have been included in governmental programs, such as Medicaid, for decades. More recently, they have also been included for reimbursement under private payment coverage plans as well. "In the U.S., certified nurse–midwives (CNMs) — registered nurses trained in midwifery — accept only low-risk patients. If problems develop, a physician is called. CNMs also provide pre- and postnatal care and reproductive health advice" (5).

Midwifery has seen a resurgence since the 1970s as mothers have increasingly become interested in natural childbirth and the more personalized care of the midwife. "Contemporary midwives attend births in hospitals and birthing centers as well as at home. Most midwives are registered nurses

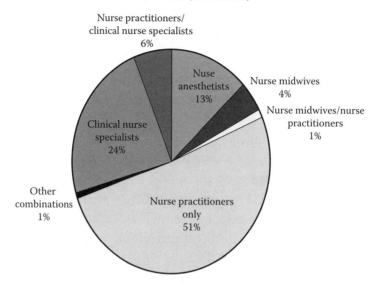

Registered Nurses Prepared for Advance Practice, 2004
Total: 240,460 RNs (8.3% of RNs)*

Nurse practitioners/
clinical nurse specialists
6%

Nuse
anesthetists
13%

Nurse midwives
4%

Nurse midwives/nurse
practitioners
1%

Clinical nurse
specialists
24%

Other
combinations
1%

Nurse practitioners
only
51%

Figure 6.4   Registered nurses prepared for advance practice: 2004. *The totals of the APN preparation distribution percents may not equal 100 percent due to the effect of rounding. This chart covers those who claimed advanced preparation as APNs in at least one specialty. Source: U.S. Department of Labor, Bureau of Labor Statistics. Occupational Employment Statistics — Registered Nurses, 2004. Accessed October 23, 2008. http://bhpr.hrsa.gov/healthworkforce/rnsurvey04/3.htm

who have completed additional training in accredited institutions. Certified nurse midwives (CNMs) can practice in all 50 states. Many are trained to deal with other gynecological issues, such as birth control and menopausal problems. Lay-midwives usually train by apprenticeship and are regulated by local statutes that limit what services they may perform" (5).

Nurse anesthetists are found in hospital and ambulatory surgery sites performing anesthetic services for a wide range of surgical and diagnostic procedures. Nurse anesthetists or certified RN anesthetists (CRNAs) work as licensed independent practitioners or, depending on state law in individual states, may require some degree of direct supervision from the physician or surgeon who is performing the operation at the time. None of these state laws requires supervision by an anesthesiologist.

CRNAs practice in all 50 states of the United States and administer approximately 30 million anesthetics each year (AANA 2006 Practice Profile Survey). For their training, nurse anesthetists complete a four-year baccalaureate degree in nursing or a science-related subject and must successfully complete the licensing examination to become an RN. Prior to entering a specialized graduate-level program in nursing anesthesia, the nurse is required to gain at least one year of clinical experience in an acute care setting, such as medical intensive care unit or surgical intensive care unit (some schools require two or more years of clinical experience). Having gained the necessary experience, nurse applicants are eligible to enroll in an accredited program of anesthesia education for an additional two to three years during which they will receive a combination of intensive theory, didactic education, and clinical practice. Finally, in order to gain the designation of CRNA, the nurse must pass a mandatory national certification examination.

CRNAs remain the highest compensated of all nursing specialties. Their average reported annual salary range in 2007, reported by the AMGA Medical Group Compensation and Financial Survey, was $140,013 (6).

6.3.4 Nurse Practitioners

As APNs, NPs also complete a master's degree in nursing. There are just fewer than 150,000 NPs in the United States currently. They work in a variety of primary care and hospital settings performing such patient care services as physical exams, diagnosis and treatment of acute illnesses and injuries, immunizations, chronic disease management, patient education, and ordering/interpreting tests. NPs are authorized to prescribe medications in all 50 states, and they can practice independently without physician collaboration or supervision in 25 states. The recent dramatic growth of mini clinics has been possible through the employment of NPs who are typically the sole clinical professional seeing and treating patients in this setting.

6.3.5 Clinical Nurse Specialists

CNSs work primarily in the hospital providing care in areas such as cardiac, oncology, obstetrics/gynecology, pediatrics, neurology, and mental health. They are also found in clinics, nursing homes, private offices, and community-based settings. CNSs also teach in nursing education programs, an area where the lack of faculty is a barrier to expanding the training of nurses to fill the shortages that were discussed above. There are just more than 70,000 CNSs in the United States (7).

6.3.6 *Licensed Practical Nurses*

Licensed practical nurses (LPNs) or licensed vocational nurses (LVNs) work generally at the bedside or in physician practices and are found in hospitals and in settings such as long-term care and home care. An LPN, also called a licensed vocational nurse in some states, will have completed a 12- to 14-month post–high school educational course that focuses on basic nursing care. In the current environment of a high demand for nursing personnel, some high schools are designing curricula that prepare the individual to successfully complete a brief period of study or even to directly complete the licensing examination upon graduation from high school. In order to become an LPN, the individual must pass the NCLEX-PN licensing examination. In 2005, there were about 710,000 LPNs in the United States with an average salary of $36,210 (4).

6.4 Physicians Assistants

Physician assistants (PAs) (8) practice medicine with a substantial level of independence but under the supervision of physicians and surgeons. The almost 80,000 PAs in the United States have been formally trained to provide diagnostic, therapeutic, and preventive healthcare services. Working as members of the healthcare team, they take medical histories, examine and treat patients, order and interpret laboratory tests and x-rays, and make diagnoses and prescribe medications. They also treat minor injuries by suturing, splinting, and casting.

While PAs work under the supervision of a licensed physician, in some poor-access areas such as remote rural areas or clinics, PAs are the only medical provider in the area. In these situations, they may work under the minimal direct supervision of a physician who may spend only brief periods in the office or clinic in which the PA works. In all cases, the PA consults with the licensed physician as needed in complex cases that call on diagnostic and treatment skills beyond those for which the PA is licensed.

PAs are trained in the medical model of education that includes both didactic learning in the classroom and application in the clinical or hospital setting. Most PA educational programs require the student applicant to complete at least two years of undergraduate education with the inclusion of premedicine courses such as biology and chemistry in the curriculum. They then go on to PA training programs that typically last for 24 to 30 months.

In total, they have at least four years of college education. As of 2007, there were 136 education programs for PAs that are accredited or provisionally accredited by the American Academy of Physician Assistants (8). Before going into practice, all PAs are required to pass the Physician Assistant National Certifying Examination in order to be licensed by their state or the District of Columbia.

6.4.1 Pharmacists

There are about 250,000 pharmacists in the United States. Of these, about 60% work in retail pharmacies, most of which are owned by major corporate chains throughout the country. About 25% of pharmacists work in hospital pharmacies, and the balance work in research, in government organizations, with payer plans, or in other related pharmaceutical fields (p. 205) (9).

In the hospital, the pharmacist supports the medication needs of both inpatients and outpatients. With the publication of the Institute of Medicine reports *To Err is Human* and *Crossing the Chasm*, the role of pharmacists has expanded. The Institute of Medicine reported that 98,000 deaths that occur in U.S. hospitals each year are due to preventable errors. A substantial portion of these deaths are due to medication errors. With this revelation, the work of pharmacists became focused not only on dispensing medications but also on the process of medication management and error reduction. This has entailed pharmacist involvement and leadership in the development and implementation of information systems for computerized provider order entry, for bar coding of medications, for medication management systems, and for the training and workflow change of everyone in the process chain of medication administration, from the physician to the nurse to the pharmacist.

The pharmacist's role, both in retail pharmacies and in hospitals, is also transforming in response to the increased demand for patient education and patient counseling, and this has become a core part of the role of pharmacists. They can expect their role to continue to evolve as the population ages and as the availability of new pharmaceuticals offers more and more opportunities for physicians and their patients to address medical problems through noninvasive means.

As described by the American Pharmacy Association, "contemporary hospital pharmacy practice is composed of a number of highly specialized areas, including nuclear pharmacy, drug and poison information, and intravenous therapy. In addition, pharmacists provide specialized services in adult medicine, pediatrics, oncology, ambulatory care, and psychiatry." (10) The nature and size of the hospital help determine the extent to which these specialized services are needed. Because of the diversity of activities involved in pharmacy departments, there is also an increasing demand for management expertise, including finance and budgeting, personnel administration, systems development, and planning.

Outside of the retail pharmacy setting, approximately 38,000 registered pharmacists work on a full- or part-time basis in hospitals or nursing homes. "As hospital pharmacists continue to become more involved in providing patient-oriented services, the demand for practitioners in this area of pharmacy continues to grow. Recent years have also seen dramatic growth in pharmacy services in health maintenance organizations (HMO) and related organizations that offer coordinated ambulatory care by a multidisciplinary staff of health professionals, including pharmacists. In this setting, pharmacists provide primary leadership in the development of both clinical and administrative systems which manage and improve the use of medications" (10).

Pharmacists are also finding a new role relative to the management of chronic diseases. In some states, in fact, pharmacists have been given authority to "initiate or modify drug treatment, as long as they have collaborative agreements with physicians. For example, a patient who need[s] blood-thinning medication might walk into the drugstore for an assessment and walk out with a different dosage of the medication that he/she has been taking" (p. 134) (11).

Pharmacy education varies slightly from school to school. All schools of pharmacy offer the PharmD degree, which requires six years of education. In pursuing this education, the student will be provided both the didactic experience of the classroom and the interactive experience of working in practice internships. Upon completion of their PharmD, the aspiring pharmacist must complete a licensing examination called the North American Pharmacist Licensure Examination™ (NAPLEX®), which is administered by the National Association of Boards of Pharmacy. This examination is accepted in all states except California, which administers its own licensing examination (10).

6.4.2 Other Allied Health Professionals

While nursing by sheer numbers is the largest single clinical profession in the hospital or health system, many other licensed and certified professionals comprise the aggregate field of what are called "allied health professionals."

Throughout the hospital, there are a number of licensed personnel who do not necessarily work at the bedside, and so are not visible to the patient, but are nonetheless essential to the services that are performed for the patient. These professionals include medical technologists who work in the laboratory performing the many types of laboratory tests on bodily fluids and tissues that are ordered for diagnostic purposes. The accuracy of their work is key to accurate diagnosis. The medical technologist works under the supervision of a director (or any other related position) of laboratory services and under oversight of a pathologist, if the department director is not a pathologist. He or she is supported by medical laboratory technicians who are prepared through a two-year associate degree. The medical technologist, on the other hand, must complete four years of college-level training in clinical laboratory science, which includes several years of classroom study and at least one year of clinical internship rotations. While a number of states require the medical technologist to complete a licensing examination in order to practice, most states seek documentation that the technologist is certified by the American Society of Clinical Pathologists. With this certification, they carry the designation of "MT" after their names.

6.4.3 Radiology Technologists

Radiology technologists are the professionals who staff the x-ray services at hospitals, health systems, ambulatory centers, diagnostic radiology centers, and other such sites. According to the Bureau of Labor Statistics, the field of radiology technology is expected to be the fastest growing of all occupations. Employment of radiology technologists is expected to increase by 15% from 2006 to 2016 (1).

The responsibility of radiology technologists is composed of preparing the equipment and patients for radiology exams and for providing the images to radiologists and physicians who ordered the tests. All radiology images are reviewed by a physician who specializes in radiology (radiologist) but are also frequently used directly by the ordering physician for diagnosis.

Radiology technologists are prepared for their profession typically through four years of college education that, similarly to that for laboratory technologists, is composed of several years in the classroom and rotation or internship in a radiology department. They may be certified by the American Registry of Radiologic Technologists, and this certification and/or licensure is required by many states and by employers. With the increased development of radiologic procedures and equipment and the use of radiology in the treatment of cancer (radiation of tumorous growths), radiologic technologists have the opportunity to specialize in their field. They are supported by radiology technicians, whose training at the associate degree level or below prepared them to perform basic x-ray procedures and to prepare films and equipment for the technologist, as well as to perform other supportive functions in the department such as helping patients to the examination room and preparing them for the procedure.

While the demand for radiology technologists continues to grow and there are about 600 training programs available to them, the supply of licensed professionals is not keeping pace with demand (12). Professionals in this field tend to earn less than their counterparts in other clinical areas, so the attractiveness of the field is diminished by the potential for a higher income elsewhere.

6.4.4 Physical, Occupational, and Speech Therapists

Physical, occupational, and speech therapists are also found in the hospital that offers a rehabilitation unit as well as in private practice and in independent, freestanding rehabilitation centers. Each of these therapists focuses on a different area of recuperative specialty.

"Physical therapists provide services that help restore function, improve mobility, relieve pain, and prevent or limit permanent physical disabilities of patients suffering from injuries or disease. They restore, maintain, and promote overall fitness and health. Their patients include accident victims and individuals with disabling conditions such as low-back pain, arthritis, heart disease, fractures, head injuries, and cerebral palsy" (13).

Educationally, physical therapists are master's degree prepared in a program that requires both classroom didactic study and practical application in a clinical setting. Upon receiving a master's degree from an accredited program and prior to entering into practice, the physical therapist graduate must successfully complete the national examination and acquire a license to practice in his or her state of choice.

The title of "speech therapist" is self-explanatory of the work of the professional. Also known as speech–language pathologists, speech therapists work with people who have any of an array of speech disorders. They work not only in hospitals: many are found in schools and in other settings in which a speech disorder may be diagnosed early and corrected. Each professional in this field requires a master's degree and must pass a national certification examination.

The registered occupational therapist (OTR) works with the patient to help him or her regain the ability to perform activities of daily living, such as cooking, driving, bathing, working with the computer, and so on.(p. 141) (11). While many of the occupational therapists in the field today may have graduated with a four-year college degree, currently all OTRs complete a minimum of a master's degree in 1 of the 124 master's degree programs available to them. As with other clinical professionals, OTRs are required to successfully complete the national examination for certification, and in order to be eligible to do so, students must complete at least two supervised clinical internships in physical disabilities, pediatrics, or mental health. Upon successful completion of the internships, graduates must pass a national examination (National Board for Certification in Occupational Therapy) before entering practice, and in all states in the United States, they are required to be licensed (14).

6.5   Other Allied Health Professionals

Within the healthcare provider setting is a wide range of other allied health professionals, many of whom work behind the scenes of direct patient care. They include registered dietitians, social workers, audiologists, psychologists, recreation therapists, and others.

6.5.1 Supporting Professionals

Hospitals and health systems cannot function without other nonclinical professionals, many of whom also work behind the scenes of patient care. These include the engineers whose attention is on the buildings and facilities; environmental specialists whose focus is on the cleanliness and orderliness of the facilities; safety managers who address hazards for employees, patients, and others; financial professionals whose role is in accounting, billing, and other financial functions; supply managers who ensure that clinical, food, environmental, and other supplies are on hand and available as needed; and administrative professionals in management, marketing, human resources, information technology, community relations, planning, facility development, fundraising, and other key roles. Additionally, others work directly with patients in roles such as those of care coordinators, chaplains, and social workers. These roles are found not only in hospitals; many of them are also in nursing care facilities, specialty services, large physician practices, and networks of providers of care.

6.5.2 Researchers

Researchers have a key role to play in healthcare. They are found in academic medical centers and in teaching hospitals, in pharmaceutical and other vendor companies, and in government. They work at the forefront of finding and developing new drugs, procedures, and technologies that advance medical care. Within the community of researchers are physicians, nurses, and other scientists. As researchers in medical science, these professionals are often required to undertake human clinical trials to test new drugs and technologies. When this is the case, they are required to obtain the approval of an institutional review board (IRB). An institutional review board exists in U.S. research institutions to ensure that research of any kind involving humans is done within defined ethical standards.

6.6   Shortage of Clinical Personnel in the United States

The United States currently faces a shortage of medical personnel in many of the clinical professions. In the 2007 Survey of Hospital Leaders, the American Hospital Association learned that there were about 116,000 registered nursing vacancies in healthcare. This represents an 8.1% shortage. Additionally, there were an 11.4% shortage among speech, occupational, and physical therapists and an 8.1% shortage among pharmacists. In response to these and a much wider anticipated gap in clinical positions in the next 10 years, some hospitals have opened new nursing programs, universities have initiated or expanded programs in the clinical professions, and some hospitals have continued the practice of looking to other countries to recruit personnel, particularly nurses.

According to the study by the American Hospital Association, 17% of hospitals reported that they hire foreign-educated nurses — 84% saying that their recruitment takes place in the Philippines. To a lesser extent, Canada, India, Ghana, Nigeria, and Zimbabwe are the prime targets for nurse recruitment (15). However, there is growing concern about this phenomenon of international recruiting. As one country draws trained personnel from another, that country finds itself facing shortages — this is particularly devastating in countries that are underserved. While the more developed country gains the benefit of expanding its workforce with foreign-educated nurses, the underdeveloped country that has invested in their education experiences worsening shortages.

Other strategies are also being pursued to expand the clinical workforce including primarily the expansion of training programs in the United States; however, other issues must also be addressed in order to find a long-term solution. What is perceived by nursing and allied health professionals as inadequate compensation, long work hours, and a stressful work environment on the one hand, and more lucrative opportunities on the other, are key challenges to be addressed in solving the critical shortage that the country faces.

6.6.1 *Administrative Management Professionals*

Finally, a discussion of the professionals in the healthcare provider workforce would not be complete without the inclusion of those whose responsibility it is to set the direction for the healthcare enterprise and manage and direct it organizationally so that all the elements work together coherently and efficiently. The field of healthcare management is responsible for providing leadership, strategic vision, structure, and direction to organizations that are very complex. While we have been discussing the internal clinical arena of the hospital or health system as the focus of the professions mentioned in this chapter, the C-suite (CEO, COO, CFO, CIO, CMO, CNO, etc.) of administrative professionals is also responsible for directing and managing the organization's relationship with the external environment. That environment imposes extensive federal, state, and local legislation on the organization; a public that is demanding; payer organizations with whom the administrators must negotiate reimbursement rates and financing mechanisms; vendors of the thousands of products used in the healthcare system each day; governance structures; competitors; and economic and environmental forces that impact the business of the organization.

Administrators in healthcare provider organizations are generally educationally prepared in master's programs in health administration. These programs are found in a variety of academic settings, including schools of medicine, of public health, business administration and allied health sciences. Persons entering the field of health administration public admistrations at an entry level may be prepared in a bachelor's degree program; however, an advanced degree is typically required in order for them to enter the ranks of upper management. In addition to the MHA, degrees such as the MPH (master;s of public health), MHSA (master.s of health services administration), and MBA (master's of business administration) are seen among the senior management ranks.

6.7.1 Nursing Facility Adminstration

The requirement for practice as a nursing home administrator is quite different from that as the hospital administrator. Nursing home administrators may come from any of a number of educational programs and may have clinical or management experience. While they do not have a defined educational requirement in most states, nursing home administrators are required to pass a licensing examination in order to be licensed in the state in which the facility is located. This examination is typically administered by the National Association of Boards of Examiners of Long-Term Care Administrators. Some states require a bachelor's degree or other formal education, however, many states do not.

6.8   Summary

Healthcare is composed of a wide array of clinicians and nonclinical professionals. Their training is extensive, and the opportunity for career growth is expansive. Their professions require that they complete rigorous education programs and successfully complete a licensure examination in the state in which they practice. While the United States continues to expand its educational opportunities for the various clinical professions, the country faces a near-term shortage of many nurses and other clinicians. A solution to that shortage is one that will require creativity, funding, and expansion of training programs if it is to be addressed effectively. The historical approach of recruiting from other countries only to leave them bereft of the workforce to meet their own needs is increasingly frowned upon in the global community.

References

1. Bureau of Labor Statistics, U.S. Department of Labor Statistics. *Occupational Outlook Handbook, 2008–2009 Edition:* "Nurses." Accessed December 2008. Available at: http://stats.bls.gov/OCO/OCOS083.HTM#projections_data and http://www.bls.gov/oco/ocos083.htm

2. L. Aiken, S. Clarke, D. Sloane, et al., 2002. "Hospital nurse staffing and patient mortality, nurse burnout, and job dissatisfaction." *Journal of American Medical Association*, 288(16):1987–1993.

3. United States General Accounting Office, 2001. "Nursing Workforce: Emerging Nurse Shortage Due to Multiple Factors." GAO-01-944. Accessed December 2008. Available at: http://www.gao.gov/new.items/d01944.pdf

4. American Nurses Association, 2007. "About Nursing." Accessed December 2008. Available at: http://www.nursingworld.org/MainMenuCategories/CertificationandAccreditation/AboutNursing.aspx

5. Britannica Concise Encyclopedia, Answers Corporation, 2008. "Nurse Midwives." Available at: http://www.answers.com/topic/nurse-midwife

6. **American Medical Group Association,** 2007. **"**Medical Group Compensation and Financial Survey, 2007 AMGA MID-LEVEL COMPENSATION." Accessed December 2008. Available at: http://www.cejkasearch.com/compensation/amga_midlevel_compensation_survey.htm

7. **American Association of Colleges of Nurses. Accessed December 2008. Available at: http://www.aacn.nche.edu/**

8. Bureau of Labor Statistics, U.S. Department of Labor Statistics. *Occupational Outlook Handbook, 2008–2009 Edition*: "Physicians Assistants." Accessed December 2008. Available at: http://www.bls.gov/oco/ocos081.htm

9. H. A. Sultz and K. M. Young (2009). *Health Care USA: Understanding Its Organization and Delivery.* Jones and Bartlett Publishers: Sudbury, MA. p. 205

10. American Pharmacists Association (2008). Accessed December 2008. Available at: http://www.pharmacist.com/AM/Template.cfm?Section=Search1&template=/CM/HTMLDisplay.cfm&ContentID=3553

11. L. Shi and D. A. Singh (2001). *Delivering Health Care in America: A Systems Approach, 2nd Edition*. Aspen Publishers: Gaithersburg, MD. pp. 134–141

12. Bureau of Labor Statistics, U.S. Department of Labor Statistics. *Occupational Outlook Handbook, 2008–2009 Edition*: "Radiologic Technologists and Technicians." Accessed December 2008. Available at: http://www.bls.gov/oco/ocos105.htm#nature

13. Bureau of Labor Statistics, U.S. Department of Labor Statistics. *Occupational Outlook Handbook, 2008–2009 Edition*: "Physical Therapists." Accessed December 2008. Available at: http://www.bls.gov/oco/ocos080.htm

14. Bureau of Labor Statistics, U.S. Department of Labor Statistics. *Occupational Outlook Handbook, 2008–2009 Edition*: "Occupational Therapists." Accessed December 2008. Available at: http://www.bls.gov/oco/ocos078.htm

15. E. Ea, 2007. "Facilitating acculturation of foreign-educated nurses." *OJIN: Online Journal of Issues in Nursing*, 13(1). Available at: http://www.nursingworld.org/MainMenuCategories/ANAMarketplace/ANAPeriodicals/OJIN/TableofContents/vol132008/No1Jan08/ArticlePreviousTopic/ForeignEducatedNurses.aspx

Chapter 7

The Legal and Regulatory Environment

7.1 Introduction

The government's role in healthcare delivery is threefold. The government serves as a *payer* of healthcare, as a *provider* of healthcare, and as a *regulator* of healthcare. Each of these roles is distinct, and each has its own impact on the delivery of healthcare.

At the federal level, the government serves as a payer of healthcare through programs such as Medicare, Medicaid, the Veterans Administration, the Indian Health Services, and other such structures. State governments are also payers of healthcare through their administration and funding of Medicaid, the State Children's Health Insurance Program, mental health services, and public health services. Likewise, local governments participate in both paying for and providing healthcare services through their financial support and/or ownership of screening, diagnostic, and treatment clinics and for hospitals owned and operated by the county or city.

In its role as a provider of healthcare, the government owns and operates direct service departments such as the Veterans Administration through veterans hospitals and the Indian Health Services, which are owned and administered by the government and through state-operated mental health facilities and hospitals that a number of counties in various states own and operate (e.g., Grady Health System in Atlanta owned by the Fulton-DeKalb Hospital Authority, John H. Stroger, Jr. Hospital of Cook County in Chicago).

The role of regulator is the one we tend to recognize first when we think of the government in healthcare. A plethora of laws and regulations control and direct the ways and methods by which healthcare is delivered from the most basic issues of cleanliness to the more complex areas of financing and technology.

In this chapter, we address primarily the role of government as regulator. Its role as payer will come into the discussion in chapter 8 on financing of healthcare. Its role as provider was discussed in chapter 3 on the structures of healthcare delivery providers.

7.1.1 The Government as Regulator

The government regulates healthcare in a wide variety of areas, as mentioned above, from the most basic realms of cleanliness for infection control to the more complex realms of capital financing mechanisms and the performance of highly sophisticated medical procedures. As regulator, the impact of governmental requirements comes not only from the legislative branch but also from the executive and judicial branches. The legislative branch puts laws in place, the executive branch implements those laws and issues detailed regulations that guide their implementation, and the judicial branch issues decisions that have the impact of law in their interpretation. In this chapter, we discuss some of the major laws and regulations that shape the way in which healthcare has been and is delivered in the United States.

Within the executive branch of the government, the Department of Health and Human Services holds primary responsibility for the implementation of statutes regulating healthcare. See chapter 11, Public Health, for an organizational chart and a description of the various departments and agencies of the federal government.

7.2   The Legislature: Healthcare Statutes

While a plethora of laws have converged upon healthcare providers over the past centuries, this discussion will focus on a number of the laws of the past several decades that continue to have a major and widespread impact on healthcare. For a comprehensive review of healthcare legislation, go to www.healthlawyers.com. Table 7.1 provides a partial list of major legislative initiatives affecting healthcare in the United States since 1946. Several of them are discussed below.

Table 7.1 Chronology of Major Healthcare Legislation in the United States

1946	Hospital Survey and Construction Act (Hill-Burton Act), PL 79-725
1949	Hospital Construction Act, PL 81-380
1950	Public Health Services Act Amendments, PL 81-692
1955	Poliomyelitis Vaccination Assistance Act, PL 84-377
1956	Health Research Facilities Act, PL 84-835
1960	Social Security Amendments (Kerr-Mill Aid), PL 86-778
1961	Community Health Services and Facilities Act, PL 87-395
1962	Public Health Service Act, PL 87-838 Vaccination Assistance, PL 87-868
1963	Mental Retardation Facilities Construction Act/Community Mental Health Centers Act, PL 88-164
1964	Nurse Training Act, PL 88-581
1965	Community Health Services and Facilities Act, PL 89-109
	Medicare and Medicaid, PL 89-97
	Mental Health Centers Act Amendments, PL 89-105
	Heart Disease, Cancer, and Stroke Amendments, PL 89-239
1966	Comprehensive Health Planning and Service Act, PL 89-749
1970	Community Mental Health Service Act, PL 91-211
	Family Planning Services and Population Research Act, PL 91-572
	Lead-Based Paint Poisoning Prevention Act, PL 91-695
1971	National Cancer Act, PL 92-218
1973	Health Maintenance Organization Act, PL 93-222
1974	Research on Aging Act, PL 93-296
	National Health Planning and Resources Development Act (Created CON), PL 93-641
1979	Department of Education Organization Act (Created HHS), PL 96-88
1982	Tax Equity and Fiscal Responsibility Act (TEFRA), PL 97-248
1983	Amendments to the Social Security Act (Prospective Payment System), PL 106-113
1985	Consolidated Omnibus Reconciliation Act (COBRA), PL 99-272
1987	Department of Transportation Appropriations Act, PL 100-202
	Omnibus Budget Reconciliation Act (OBRA), PL 100-203
1988	Medicare Catastrophic Coverage Act, PL 100-360
1989	Department of Transportation and Related Agencies Appropriations Act, PL 101-164
1993	Family and Medical Leave Act, PL 103-3
1996	Health Insurance Portability and Accountability Act, PL 104-191
1997	Balanced Budget Act (BBA), PL 105-33
2002	Public Health Security and Bioterrorism Preparedness and Response Act, PL 107-188
2005	Patient Safety and Quality Improvement Act, PL 109-41

7.2.1 Hill-Burton

After World War II, the United States found itself in a position in which health insurance was being made available through employers, but many people were being denied access to hospitals because there were not enough beds in which to house them. With a report on hand from the Commission on Hospital Care (1) indicating a need for 195,000 beds across the country, particularly in poorer and rural areas, U.S. Senators Lister Hill (D-AL) and Harold Burton (R-OH) sponsored the Hospital Survey and Construction Act in 1946, which came to be known in healthcare parlance as the Hill-Burton Act. The legislation was intended to fund the development of new and replacement hospitals in underserved areas across the country. Its initial 5-year commitment of $75 million in funding was extended into subsequent years, until within 20 years it had funded "nearly 8,200 construction and expansion projects that provided an estimated 349,318 beds" (1). The Hill-Burton Act was still funding hospital construction in the 1970s.

The building boom that was generated by the Hill-Burton program carried a proviso for each of the hospitals that received funding under it. That proviso required the hospital to provide assurance that it would be available to the community in perpetuity and that it would provide charity care. However, the level of charity care was not defined, nor was there a time limit on it, and it was not until court cases and regulatory actions in the 1960s and 1970s that the time commitment for the provision of charity care was established under a 20-year time frame.

In the current context of the early twenty-first century, it is important to understand the impact of Hill-Burton on healthcare today. Under this program, hospital capacity in the United States expanded dramatically. Many small communities came to have "their own" hospital, and they took pride in the presence of a hospital in their communities. Doctors were more willing to move to small communities knowing they would have a hospital in which to care for their acute care patients, perform surgical procedures, and birth babies. While this sense of security and expansion prevailed, there was no control on the fees that insurers paid for services in the hospitals or doctors' offices. To the contrary, more expansion of government financing was at hand through Medicare and Medicaid. After 20 years of building hospitals throughout the country, a heightened awareness developed of the number of people who could not access those hospitals because they did not have the wherewithal to pay for services. In rural communities, it was the poor and the elderly who comprised a large proportion of the population. As they sought medical care and did not have the means to pay, hospitals became concerned about their financial viability. They were obliged to care for the indigent under their Hill-Burton funding, but they had not planned on the volume impact of charity care on their finances.

7.3 Medicare and Medicaid (Titles XVIII and XIX of the Social Security Amendments)

Awareness of the cost of charity care led directly to the passage of Medicare and Medicaid in the 1960s. With these programs, the operational viability of the many hospitals built under Hill-Burton was assured. While we will talk more about this later, it is an interesting point to note that both programs paid for medical care on a cost-plus basis. This means that there was no limit on the fees that Medicare would pay to hospitals. In fact, Medicare paid all costs for enrolled patients plus a 2% "profit" — the hospital could take on as much debt for construction and expansion of services and could hire as many staff as it wanted — there was no monitoring of provider costs in the early days of the Medicare Program. This lasted only a couple of years, until the costs of Medicare and Medicaid began to escalate out of control and to usher in the days of cost containment. While the passage of Medicare and Medicaid was a watershed day for healthcare in the United States, a new cost containment policy was needed.

7.3.1 Certificate of Need (1973)

A major element of that new policy was Certificate of Need (CON) — a program that is still in effect in most states. The CON requires healthcare providers to gain state approval before expansion, acquisition, or creation of new services. In each of these investments, the state has predetermined expenditure and expansion thresholds at which the healthcare provider needs to apply for a CON. That is an established capital expenditure level is in place in most states that have CON programs and providers who undertake construction or expansion costing above those thresholds, are required to apply for a CON.

While before CON the congress and administration had tried a number cost containment methods to control the spiraling costs of Medicare and Medicaid, most were to little avail in accomplishing a reversal of the dramatic cost increase trend following the implementation of Medicare and Medicaid. By the early 1970s, it was clear to the legislature that the building boom introduced by the Hill-Burton program had to be slowed and infused with planning for facilities based on population need. The cost of debt was a major expense to Medicare, but more importantly, the phenomenon of "if we build it, they will come" drove expenses beyond all budgeted expectations. Healthcare dollars spent on construction and equipment needed to be spent based on a planned determination of population need for the related health services (i.e., the need for acute care beds, nursing homes, etc.)

What ensued was passage of the Health Planning and Resources Development Act, Section 93-641 of the Social Security Act in 1973. While the statute provided for formalized planning of the services needed, the statute quickly came to be known as the "CON" law. The statute called upon each state to pass implementation laws for the establishment of planning agencies to lead the development of plans that would identify needed healthcare resources in their respective states. It also called for the review of major capital expenditures and of expansion capacity or creation of new services by healthcare providers. The new CON laws placed both civil and criminal penalties on providers of care who undertook major capital expenditures or who expanded into new services without the requisite CON approval. The intent of this law was to both limit the development of healthcare resources based on need as defined by the state and to reduce the duplication of services and thus reduce the rate of cost increase in healthcare.

The intent of the CON law was twofold: (1) to ensure that expenditures that were being made in the private and public sectors were for services needed by the community or region and to reduce the duplication of expensive facilities and services that was occurring in many areas and (2) to curb the expansion of facilities and services whose growth had been rampant under the Hill-Burton Act and under the provisions of Medicare and Medicaid in which capital costs were not constrained and were believed to be driving the rise in healthcare costs.

Under the new law, all providers were required to submit to a local review body the complete plans and the justification of the need for the expansion or new services. After completing its review, the local or regional planning body would then recommend action to a state review board whose responsibility was to take final action in determining whether or not to issue a CON for the project.

While CON became the best-known part of the Health Planning and Resources Development Act, there was another part of the act that called for the planning of health services based on population need. Under Section 93-641, states were required to create a health planning function in which analysis of population and community needs could be completed and through which each state would designate the extent of services and number of beds needed to adequately serve the population (e.g., the number of acute and long-term care beds per 1000 population and the number of open heart surgery and other tertiary services needed). The State then supported its decision relative to issuance of the CON based on its assessment of each project against the state health plan.

Much controversy swirled around many capital projects as they moved forward in the public review process. That process was open to statements and documentation from other providers in the geographic area of the applicant organization, to consumers, to employers, and to anyone from the public who wanted to have input. Thus, competitive forces were introduced into the process. Competitors, neighbors, and consumers could be vocal in support of or disagreement with applicationd project.

In 1987, PL 93-641, the federal government sunset (repeated) the CON law, and states were authorized to repeal their respective CON laws. Some did repeal their CON requirements, but 36 states, the District of Columbia, and Puerto Rico continue to maintain a CON review of capital expenditures in their states. In maintaining this barrier to entry and to expansion, existing hospitals and other providers of care are sustained within their markets, and they argue that there will be minimal expensive duplicative services in the system. Thresholds for submission (e.g., amount of capital expenditure) vary by state, and most states that retain the requirement have moved the review process to a state level and out of the responsibility of local review agencies (2). The review process requires an extensive application that documents the area-wide need for the services proposed and that assesses the financial ability to support the proposed construction or purchase.

Overall, the intended impact of CON of reducing the rate of increase in the costs of medical care in the United States was not realized as those costs continued to rise. On the other hand, CON came to serve as a barrier to entry into healthcare markets, reducing competition for existing providers. Currently, some states are studying and implementing a number of reforms in order to promote competition within their borders. For example, Connecticut no longer requires that healthcare providers obtain approval for capital expenditure projects that do not involve clinical services (e.g., parking garages) and Iowa has relaxed the rules for replacement of rural hospitals (3).

7.3.2 HMO Act (1973)

The HMO Act of 1973 is important from the perspective of the support it gave to the development of HMOs. Up until this time, HMOs were in place in various areas throughout the country; however, they were not flourishing. Because HMOs focused on primary and preventive care, on case management, and on controlling costs, the act was intended to be part of a cost-containment initiative. Its goal was to reduce healthcare costs by eliminating regulatory barriers that inhibited HMO development. Under the act, HMOs could be designated for federal qualification by meeting certain mandates related to their benefits package, open enrollment, and community rating. With that federal certification on hand, they could go to employers who had 25 or more employees to present their plan to employees. Those employees were then required to offer the HMO option to their employees. While this latter provision was eliminated in 1995, during the early years of its existence HMOs were boosted onto the U.S. healthcare "stage" in numbers and enrollments under this mandate. Although many HMOs continued to struggle due to consumer reluctance to sign on because of the restrictions they place on choice of provider, the HMO Act of 1973 gave substantial visibility to their focus on primary care and case/cost management and helped prepare the U.S. infrastructure and "psyche" for managed care in the early to mid-1990s (4).

7.3.3 Prospective Payment (1982)

Neither CON nor the HMO Act served effectively to reduce the rate of increase in healthcare costs. Costs continued to rise beyond the rate of the consumer price index. So, Congress passed, within the Tax Equity and Fiscal Responsibility Act of 1982 (also known as TEFRA), the Social Security Amendments, which called for a case-based payment system for hospital inpatient care. Under this law, hospitals are paid a set fee that is predetermined (i.e., "prospective") based on the diagnosis under which the patient is admitted.

Implemented in 1983, hospitals are reimbursed, under this act, on the basis of diagnosis-related groups or DRGs. The structure of the payment system provides for "a patient classification scheme which provides a means of relating the type of patients a hospital treats (i.e., its case mix) to the costs incurred by the hospital" in caring for those patients (5). In this structure, hospitals are paid based on predetermined rates. The diagnosis under which the patient is treated is the determining factor under which the provider is paid. If it uses excess resources over and above those that are predetermined to be needed to treat the diagnosis, the hospital does not get paid for the additional costs, and vice versa, if the hospital can treat the patient at a lower use of resources, then the hospital still gets paid the established reimbursement rate. This rate is determined based on the case mix of the hospital (i.e., the mix of patients that it serves and the acuity of their illness or injury) and on the average costs that should be required to provide needed service to address each patient's diagnosis. The establishment of the DRG reimbursement structure "ended the era — dating back to the 1920s — in which doctors' and hospitals' authority over medical practices and decision-making went virtually unquestioned" (6).

Initially, the DRG payment system applied only to hospitals and inpatient care. Ambulatory care, rehabilitation care, long-term care, and other venues were not impacted. One of the unintended consequences of the prospective payment system was to trigger a shift in care sites from the inpatient setting to these other venues. Patients who previously might have been admitted to the hospital were instead, whenever possible, referred to a non-acute care unit or provider (e.g., rehabilitation, sub-acute care, ambulatory surgical unit). Consequently, the decade following the implementation of DRGs was marked by substantial expansion in these areas — until, of course, DRG methods came to be applied to each of them in turn over the next decade. Within the Centers for Medicare and Medicaid Services (CMS), the Prospective Payment Advisory Commission is mandated to review regularly the payment system under which providers are reimbursed and to report to Congress on any changes that it advises.

The DRG system brought with it another potential unintended consequence, that of providers who might forego diagnostic or treatment procedures for a patient in favor of saving monies that they would be paid under the preset fee. TEFRA provisions called for the establishment of physician review organizations that would be established to counter this "perverse incentive" through review of quality of care and ensure that quality did not suffer as a result of the payment system.

7.3.4 Emergency Medical Treatment and Active Labor Act (1986)

The Emergency Medical Treatment and Active Labor Act (EMTALA) "is a statute which governs when and how a patient may be (1) refused treatment or (2) transferred from one hospital to another when he is in an unstable medical condition" (7).

EMTALA was passed as part of the Consolidated Omnibus Budget Reconciliation Act of 1986 and is integrated into the Social Security Act under Section 1867(a). EMTALA evolved out of the process that hospitals were frequently employing to transfer patients who did not have the ability to pay for treatment from their emergency departments to "charity" or "county" hospitals, which are supported by local taxes and which generally serve a predominant portion of the indigent population or those covered by Medicaid.

"EMTALA is primarily but not exclusively a non-discrimination statute. One would cover most of its purpose and effect by characterizing it as providing that no patient who presents with an emergency medical condition and who is unable to pay may be treated differently than patients who are covered by health insurance. That is not the entire scope of EMTALA, however; it imposes affirmative obligations which go beyond non-discrimination" (7).

The core provisions of the law cover any patient who "comes to the emergency department" requesting "examination or treatment for a medical condition" and requires that the hospital provide "an appropriate medical screening examination." If it is determined that the patient, in fact, has an emergency condition, then the hospital is obliged either to provide treatment until the patient is stabilized or transfer that patient to another hospital. That transfer may happen only under certain circumstances, such as a lack of the specialty service that the patient needs. If it is determined that he or she can only receive the needed service at another facility that has the technology and specialty-trained personnel, then the hospital may be able to transfer the patient with the consent of the receiving hospital and with the provision of appropriately medically supported transport.

"A pregnant woman who presents in active labor must, for all practical purposes, be admitted and treated until delivery is completed, unless a transfer under the statute is appropriate" (7). "In essence, then, the statute:

- imposes an affirmative obligation on the part of the hospital to provide a medical screening examination to determine whether an 'emergency medical condition' exists;
- imposes restrictions on transfers of persons who exhibit an 'emergency medical condition' or are in active labor, which restrictions may or may not be limited to transfers made for economic reasons; [and]
- imposes an affirmative duty to institute treatment if an 'emergency medical condition' does exist" (7).

7.3.5 Stark Law — The Physician Self-Referral Act (Stark I-1989 and Stark II-1993)

Named after Representative Pete Stark (D-CA), the Stark laws were passed as measures to prevent the abuse of referral arrangements by physicians. After research reports indicated that physicians were "reaping inordinate profits from Medicare because they were referring patients to their own facilities and ordering unnecessary tests" (8), Stark I was passed to constrain the ability of physicians to refer patients for tests to facilities that they themselves owned. In other words, physicians were prohibited from "referring Medicare patients to facilities with which they have a financial relationship" (8). Stark II was passed into law only four years later in order to further constrain the financial relationships between hospitals and doctors and to prevent doctors from referring to inpatient and outpatient services in hospitals in which they own an interest unless they met one of the list of exceptions provided in the law.

As healthcare evolved into the twenty-first century, the Stark laws came to be seen as a major hindrance to some of the positive initiatives that are needed to ensure quality of care and to reduce costs, such as the adoption of the Electronic Health Record (EHR). Stark III was passed in 2007 to make changes to the earlier laws.

Because the Stark laws were a major barrier to the adoption of the EHR, the rules and regulations implementing Stark were modified in 2007 in order to allow hospitals to enter into limited financial arrangements with their doctors. Under the new provisions, hospitals can support EHR implementation in the offices of doctors on their staff. These provisions require that software is integrated between the physician's office and the hospital and that there be networking and sharing of data between the physician practice and the hospital. While the physician is required to pay at least 15% of the cost of the software and the full cost of the hardware, this modification in Stark has opened the way for hospitals and physicians to develop electronic systems for the storing, accessing, and sharing of patient data. This is key to the integration of patient care across a continuum of care or wherever the patient goes in the health provider system.

7.3.6 HIPAA (1996)

"HIPAA" has been engrained into the consciousness of almost every healthcare worker in the United States. It has become a synonym for "privacy and security." Actually, HIPAA is an acronym for the Health Insurance Portability and Accountability Act of 1996 (August 21), Public Law 104-191, which amended the Internal Revenue Service Code of 1986.

HIPAA was passed in an era of economic boom (just before the "dot com bust") when unemployment was low and many people found themselves in "job lock," unable to take advantage of better jobs because a medical condition would exclude them from their new employer's coverage for one year or more. Those with preexisting medical conditions could not afford to move up in their careers by moving to a position with a new employer because employers' health plans typically excluded those with preexisting conditions for one year or more. The cost of healthcare served as a disincentive to employees who, while awaiting coverage with the new employer, would pay more in private payment for medical care and drugs than the increase in income they might enjoy in the new job — they were in job lock.

To break the hold of job lock, Congress passed the Kennedy-Kassenbaum Act, now known simply as HIPAA. Under its Title I, HIPAA provided for nondiscrimination in employee eligibility or continued eligibility to enroll for benefits under the terms of an employer group health plan without regard to health factors. If the employee was covered by the previous employer and maintained that coverage for 18 months, the new employer is required to offer the same healthcare benefits as are offered to other employees within the organization. Under Title II, the law provided for Administrative Simplification, the provision that has had significant impact on providers who use electronic data transfer. They must provide for the security of that data and the protection of patient privacy.

Under Title I, not only must the employer group health plans not discriminate against any employee in the provision of healthcare benefits, but the employee may not be charged more for coverage than other persons under the same plan in the employer organization because of health status–related factors. While the group plan may exclude certain diseases from coverage, limit coverage benefits, and place lifetime limits on coverage, the plan must do the same for all "similarly situated individuals." It may not single out one group or individual for coverage limits due to the health factors of that group or employee. In other words, coverage must apply consistently across all covered individuals who are "similarly situated" (9).

Furthermore, the new employer's health plan must give individuals credit for the length of time they had continuous health coverage before their start of work with the employer. If, for example, the employer has a 12-month wait period before coverage takes effect for new employees' preexisting conditions, if an individual had "creditable coverage" for a 12-month period before the start of employment, without a break in coverage of 63 days or more, then that coverage must be counted to reduce or eliminate the 12-month exclusion period.

Title II of HIPAA is the Administrative Simplification section of the act. This section requires

1. improved efficiency in healthcare delivery by standardizing electronic data interchange and
2. protection of confidentiality and security of health data through setting and enforcing standards (10).

HIPAA's Title II required the Department of Health and Human Services to publish new rules to ensure the development of:

1. Standardization of electronic patient health, administrative, and financial data
2. Unique health identifiers for individuals, employers, health plans, and healthcare providers
3. Security standards protecting the confidentiality and integrity of "individually identifiable health information," past, present, or future (10).

Healthcare organizations — including all healthcare providers, health plans, public health authorities, healthcare clearinghouses, and self-insured employers — as well as life insurers, information systems vendors, various service organizations, and universities that exchange healthcare data electronically are affected by HIPAA. It is a serious business for them as noncompliance makes them subject to both civil and criminal penalties. Fines can range up to $25,000 for multiple violations of the same standard in a calendar year or up to $250,000 and/or imprisonment up to 10 years for knowing misuse of individually identifiable health information.

Compliance requirements include

- Building initial organizational awareness of HIPAA
- Comprehensive assessment of the organization's privacy practices, information security systems and procedures, and use of electronic transactions
- Developing an action plan for compliance with each rule
- Developing a technical and management infrastructure to implement the plans
- Implementing a comprehensive implementation action plan, including

- developing new policies, processes, and procedures to ensure privacy, security, and patients' rights
- building business associate agreements with business partners to support HIPAA objectives
- developing a secure technical and physical information infrastructure
- updating information systems to safeguard protected health information and enable use of standard claims and related transactions
- training of all workforce members
- developing and maintaining an internal privacy and security management and enforcement infrastructure, including providing a privacy officer and a security officer (10)

7.3.7 Malpractice

While we might have discussed malpractice within the context of our discussion on physicians, it is appropriate to have that discussion here. In the litigious society of the United States, the level of legal action against physicians and, in some cases, the tens of millions of dollars in rewards have driven up the cost of malpractice insurance for physicians — to the point at which $100,000 to $150,000 premiums are not uncommon for certain specialties. More particularly, it has placed pressure on physicians to find ways in which to cover that cost.

During the 1990s, the United States experienced a particularly rapid increase in physician malpractice premiums, just as physician incomes were being curbed under RBRVS and under managed care plans. Physicians found themselves not only in the dilemma of earning less revenue in their practices but also coping with rapidly rising costs of insurance. The "epidemic" of physician response grew in states throughout the country, with some leaving the practice of medicine, others moving into new physician-related professions, and some others moving en masse out of certain states. The crises that resulted pushed states to find solutions, and different states took different courses of action. Some established their own state-operated malpractice insurance programs offering lower premiums to doctors, and others moved to tort reform, establishing ceilings on the amount of damages that plaintiffs could be awarded in malpractice cases and on the amounts of fees paid to lawyers. For a number of years, these measures "cooled" the heightened concern of the 1990s; however, from time to time and from state to state or locality to locality, issues related to the costs of malpractice insurance arise.

Medical malpractice litigation, as explained by Studdert et al., has three social goals: "to deter unsafe practices, to compensate persons injured through negligence, and to exact corrective justice" (11). Recently, an Illinois case challenging the state's cap on awards for damages is being watched carefully by hospitals, doctors, and legislatures. This is the case of *Lebron v Gottlieb Memorial Hospital,* which is under appeal to the Illinois Supreme Court. The issue in this case is whether the Illinois statutory cap on non-economic damages is constitutional under the Separation of Powers Clause of the Illinois Constitution (Ill. Const. 1970, Articles II and 1) (12).

7.4   Summary

In this chapter, we have covered only a few of the major areas of legislation and other public policy initiatives that impact healthcare providers. While this gives an overview of key statutes, it is important to consider that each of these and other laws and regulations are frequently amended or clarified through the process of regulation, of judicial decisions, and of executive orders. Additionally, since the government is a major payer of healthcare services, policy is frequently made by line items in the budgets that Congress approves and in the modifications to those line items that happen in the executive administration of the budget. Line item changes in budget allocations can, for example, provide increased or decreased support for rehabilitation while conversely increasing or decreasing support for another service, such as hospice care or home healthcare. These are the changes that happen out of the sight of the legislature, yet they have significant impact on the people who rely on the benefits of governmental payment programs and on providers who care for patients in the various specialties (e.g., in the example above, rehabilitation and hospice or home healthcare).

References

1. J. Bess, 1998. "If you build it…." *AHA News*, 7–8.
2. The National Council of State Legislatures, 2008. "Certificate of Need: State Health Laws and Programs." Accessed December 15, 2008. Available at: http://www.ncsl.org/programs/health/cert-need.htm
3. A. Robeznieks, 2008. "Feeling right at home." *Modern Healthcare*, 38(42), 36–38.

4. C. J. Conover and I. Wiechers, 2004. "HMO Act of 1973, Health Insurance Regulation Working Paper No.1.1" from *Cost of Health Services Regulation Working Paper Series*. Center for Health Policy, Law, and Management, Duke University, Durham, NC.

5. R. F. Averill, N. Goldfield, J. S. Hughes, J. Bonazelli, E. C. McCullough, B. A. Steinbeck, R. Mullin, A. M. Tang, J. Muldoon, L. Turner, and J. Gay, 2003. *All Patient Refined Diagnosis Related Groups (APR-DRGs): Methodology Overview*. 3M Health Information Systems, Wallingford, CT.

6. R. Mayes and R. Berenson, 2008. *Policymaking for Medicare: Prospective Payment and the Shaping of U.S. Health Care*. John Hopkins University Press, Baltimore, MD.

7. "Frequently Asked Questions about the Emergency Medical Transfer and Active Labor Act." Accessed December 15, 2008. Available at: http://www.emtala.com/faq.htm

8. K. Sandrick, 2008. "Stark Laws Then and Now." Trustee 61(2) 33–35.

9. Health Insurance Portability and Accountability Act of 1996 (HIPAA). *Title I — Health Care Access, Portability, and Renewability*. Accessed April 2002. Available at: http://hipaa.ohio.gov/whitepapers/title1healthcareaccess.PDF

10. "Need Help with HIPAA." Accessed December 15, 2008. Available at: http://www.hipaadvisory.com/REGS/HIPAAprimer.htm

11. D. M. Studdert, M. M. Mello, and T. A. Brennan, 2004. "Medical malpractice." *New England Journal of Medicine*, 350, 283–292.

12. "Verdict Could Derail Illinoisans' Health Care." Illinois State Medical Society. Accessed December 16, 2008. Available at: http://www.isms.org/newsroom/newsrelease/nr2007_1113.htm

Chapter 8

Financing Healthcare

8.1 Introduction

The financing of healthcare in the United States is partly public and partly private — partly "national health insurance" and partly employer sponsored, with an increasing proportion of private pay insurance and out-of-pocket payments from consumers. It is a complex system that, for all the wealth it consumes and creates in the United States, still leaves over 15% of the population with no coverage and almost another 30% with far too little coverage. It is a system that today places hospitals in the role of default insurer. They are required to accept the uninsured in their emergency departments and to provide essential diagnostic and treatment services required by the patients. This is a very expensive cost-shifting phenomenon in which costs for paying patients and insurers are increased by amounts not collected from the uninsured and underinsured. Their costs of care are included in the computation of expenses and then, inherently, in the fees that are charged to other payers.

8.2 How Much Does Healthcare Cost in the United States?

The first place to start our discussion of healthcare costs is with a focus on how much those costs are, their trends, and their distribution among the providers of care. As we ended 2006, our tab for healthcare (hospitals, physicians, pharmaceuticals, nursing home care, and so on) was $2.3 trillion or 16% of the gross domestic product (GDP). This was a rate of increase of 6.9% from the previous year (Figure 8.1) and represented a cost per person of $7,026. By 2016, healthcare expenditures are expected to reach $4.2 trillion or 20% of the GDP (1).

The United States, as compared with other countries, spends far more of its GDP on healthcare than other countries — many of which have a better overall health status than the United States (see chapter 2). Based on the most recent comparative data available, in 2004, the United States spent 15.3% of its GDP on healthcare, compared with Switzerland, the next highest spending country, which spent 11.6% of its GDP in the health sector. Farther behind Switzerland are France (10.5%), Iceland (10.2%), Canada (9.9%), and the United Kingdom (8.3%) (Figure 8.2).

Even at this level of expenditure, in 2007, there were nearly 46 million people in the United States (>15% of the population) without health insurance for at least a part of the year. According to the U.S. Census Bureau, approximately 85% of Americans have health insurance; nearly 60% obtain it through an employer, while about 9% purchase it directly (2).

Taking a closer look inside healthcare, it is informative to learn where the United States spent its healthcare dollars in 2006 (i.e., who was on the receiving end of the exchange). In 2006, hospitals were paid 31% of the

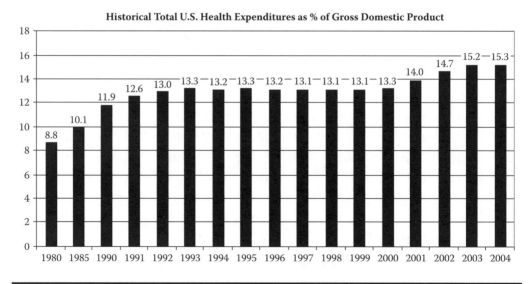

Figure 8.1   Historical total health expenditure as percentage of gross domestic product. Source: Organization for Economic Cooperation and Development, Paris, France, *OECD Health Data 2006* (copyright).

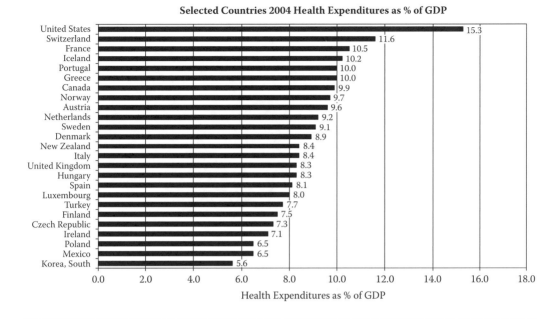

Figure 8.2   Selected countries 2004 health expenditures as percentage of GDP. Source: Organization for Economic Cooperation and Development, Paris, France, *OECD Health Data 2006* (copyright).

nation's healthcare dollar, physicians and other clinical services received 21% of the total, nursing homes received 6%, and pharmaceuticals consumed 10%. Seven percent was spent on program administration and net costs (Figure 8.3).

Before looking at each of the major programs through which public monies flow to healthcare, it is useful to gain a sense of the proportion each of these is of the nation's public national health expenditures. Figure 8.3 indicates that the majority of public expenditures are made through Medicare and that about one-third are made through Medicaid. These numbers reveal why the national focus for reductions in cost is on Medicare and Medicaid. These government-sponsored healthcare programs cover about 28% of Americans (2).

8.3   Medicare

Medicare was established under Title XVIII of the Social Security Amendments in 1965. At its outset, Medicare was created to finance care for the elderly, defined as persons aged 65 years or older. Subsequent to its

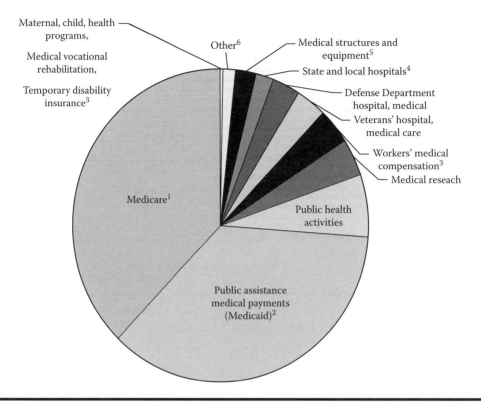

Public National Health Expenditures by Type, 2006
Total = 902.7 Billion Dollars

Figure 8.3   Public national health expenditures by type: 2006. http://www.cms.hhs. gov/NationalHealthExpendData/downloads/PieChartSourcesExpenditures2006.pdf

passage, further legislation added coverage for the disabled at any age and for persons with end-stage renal disease.

Medicare provides coverage under four distinct parts: Part A, hospital insurance or HI, covers hospital, skilled nursing, home health, and hospice care; Part B, medical insurance, pays for physician services and other medical services and supplies; Part C provides the enrollee coverage through managed care plans, such as health maintenance organizations (HMOs); and Part D provides prescription coverage. Originally, Medicare (Parts A and B) required payment premiums for Part B and of deductibles and copayments by the enrollee. These coverage exceptions are called "gaps" in Medicare, and for them, the enrollee can purchase Medicare supplemental insurance, also known as MediGap insurance, from insurers who follow federal guidelines and clearly indicate what these policies are. Each of the four parts of Medicare is described in some detail in Figure 8.4.

Medicare was born out of the 1945 vision of President Harry Truman when he proposed that the United States institute a universal healthcare program. Strongly opposed by the American Medical Association, it was not until after Lyndon Johnson took office that a more limited version of national health insurance would pass — a national health insurance package for two major sectors of society, the elderly and the indigent with Medicare and Medicaid, respectively.

Medicare Parts A, B, C, D

Part A: Hospital insurance

- Helps pay for inpatient care in a hospital or skilled nursing facility (following a hospital stay), some home health care and hospice care.

Before age 65, you are eligible for free Medicare hospital insurance if:

- You have been entitled to Social Security disability benefits for 24 months; or
- You receive a disability pension from the railroad retirement board and meet certain conditions; or
- You have Lou Gehrig's disease (amyotrophic lateral sclerosis); or
- You worked long enough in a government job where Medicare taxes were paid and you meet the requirements of the Social Security disability program; or
- You are the child or widow(er) age 50 or older, including a divorced widow(er), of someone who has worked long enough in a government job where Medicare taxes were paid and you meet the requirements of the Social Security disability program.
- You have permanent kidney failure and you receive maintenance dialysis or a kidney transplant and:
  - You are eligible for or receive monthly benefits under Social Security or the railroad retirement system; or
  - You have worked long enough in a Medicare-covered government job; or
  - You are the child or spouse (including a divorced spouse) of a worker (living or deceased) who has worked long enough under Social Security or in a Medicare-covered government job.

Part B: Medical insurance

- Helps pay for doctors' services and many other medical services and supplies that are not covered by hospital insurance.

Anyone who is eligible for free Medicare hospital insurance (Part A) can enroll in Medicare medical insurance (Part B) by paying a monthly premium. Some beneficiaries with higher incomes will pay a higher monthly Part B premium.

Figure 8.4   Medicare parts A–D. Source: Social Security Administration. SSA Publication No. 05-10043, ICN 460000. May 2008. http://www.ssa.gov/pubs/10043.pdf

Figure 8.4 Medicare parts A–D. (*Continued*)

If you are not eligible for free hospital insurance, you can buy medical insurance, without having to buy hospital insurance, if you are age 65 or older and you are—

• A U.S. citizen; or

• A lawfully admitted noncitizen who has lived in the United States for at least five years.

Part C: Medicare Advantage

• Plans are available in many areas. People with Medicare Parts A and B can choose to receive all of their health care services through one of these provider organizations under Part C.

If you have Medicare Parts A and B, you can join a Medicare Advantage plan. With one of these plans, you do not need a Medigap policy, because Medicare Advantage plans generally cover many of the same benefits that a Medigap policy would cover, such as extra days in the hospital after you have used the number of days that Medicare covers.

Medicare Advantage plans include:

• Medicare managed care plans;

• Medicare preferred provider organization (PPO) plans;

• Medicare private fee-for-service plans; and

• Medicare specialty plans.

If you decide to join a Medicare Advantage plan, you use the health card that you get from your Medicare Advantage plan provider for your health care. Also, you might have to pay a monthly premium for your Medicare Advantage plan because of the extra benefits it offers.

Part D: Prescription drug coverage

• Helps pay for medications doctors prescribe for treatment.

Anyone who has Medicare hospital insurance (Part A), medical insurance (Part B), or a Medicare Advantage plan (Part C) is eligible for prescription drug coverage (Part D). Joining a Medicare prescription drug plan is voluntary, and you pay an additional monthly premium for the coverage. You can wait to enroll in a Medicare Part D plan if you have other prescription drug coverage but, if you don't have prescription coverage that is, on average, at least as good as Medicare prescription drug coverage, you will pay a penalty if you wait to join later. You will have to pay this penalty for as long as you have Medicare prescription drug coverage.

Source: **Social Security Administration. SSA Publication No. 05-10043, ICN 460000. May 2008. http://www.ssa.gov/pubs/10043.pdf**

Administratively, Medicare was placed under the operational control of the Health Care Financing Administration within the Department of Health, Education, and Welfare. These offices later evolved into the current Centers for Medicare and Medicaid Services (CMS) within the Department of Health and Human Services.

Medicare has evolved substantially since its inception. Early on, it was expanded to provide coverage for the disabled of any age and for persons with end-stage renal disease. Initially, reimbursements to hospitals were based on costs (as defined by the hospital), with no cost control and a 2% profit margin. Hospitals billed whatever costs they incurred relative to Medicare patients, and the Medicare program paid that amount plus 2%. The 2% was meant to provide a small profit margin for investment in service development and other needs of the hospital. This was a "bonanza" to hospitals. They could hire staff to whatever levels they wanted, could build and incur debt to the level of their appetite for building and expansion, and could perform whatever procedures the doctors ordered with minimal oversight.

Under its initial reimbursement arrangement, the national Medicare budget blossomed far beyond levels anticipated by the legislature. In fact, while the implementation of the law in 1966 was budgeted for $1.8 billion, by 1970, expenditures had quadrupled to greater than $7.6 billion. Since then, Medicare expenditures have grown dramatically to greater than $400 billion in 2005. In that time, the number of Medicare enrollees has grown from the initial 19 million people to almost 45 million in 2008 (3). The growth in Medicare expenditures since its inception is shown in Figure 8.5.

Over the years since the inception of Medicare, a number of major initiatives have been taken to reduce the rate of increase in Medicare costs. Cost containment initiatives of the early 1970s were generally unsuccessful. Then, in 1974, the Health Resources and Development Act was enacted, giving birth to the Certificate of Need to control capital expenditures. The rate of increase did not abate, and in a further effort to curb rising healthcare costs, the mid-1980s saw the development of the prospective payment system (PPS), which has been described as "the single most influential postwar innovation in medical financing" (4,5). PPS "was introduced by the federal government in October, 1983, as a way to change hospital behavior through financial incentives that encourage more cost-efficient management of medical care. Under PPS, hospitals are paid a predetermined fixed rate for each Medicare admission. Each patient is classified into a Diagnosis Related Group (DRG) on the basis of clinical information. Except for certain patients

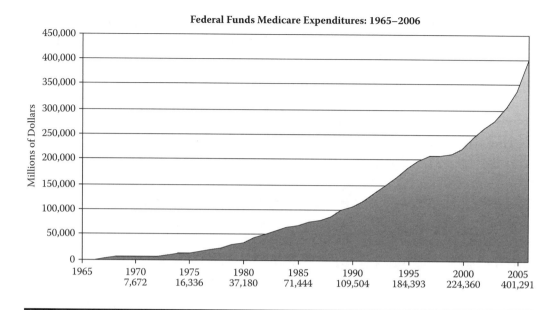

Figure 8.5　Federal funds Medicare expenditures: 1965–2006. Source: January 2008. Office of the Actuary, Centers for Medicare and Medicaid Services, historical data on national health expenditures, as published January 2008. Accessed September 2008 from, http://www.cms.hhs.gov/NationalHealthExpendData/02_ NationalHealthAccountsHistorical.asp#TopOfPage

with exceptionally high costs (called "outliers"), the hospital is paid a flat rate for the DRG, regardless of the actual services provided" (6).

Initially, the PPS was legislated and put in place with a primary focus on providers of inpatient acute care. It was not until more than 10 years later that all providers of care (ambulatory care, long-term nursing facilities, rehabilitation care) came under the prospective payment reimbursement structure. In the intervening years, care was shifted from the inpatient hospital setting to nonacute venues of care delivery for which reimbursement was not so restricted. For example, where previously a patient might have been kept in the acute care setting for a short period of recovery after a stroke, surgery, or injury, that patient was transferred to the rehabilitation unit of the hospital or to the subacute care unit of a nursing facility. Patients who previously were admitted for surgery found themselves undergoing surgery in an outpatient surgical setting, the growth of which was spurred by technological advances such as the laser and minimally invasive endoscopic surgery. Figure 8.6 reflects just how rapidly outpatient or ambulatory visits increased and how inpatient admissions decreased between 1983 and 1995.

The financial viability or sustainability of Medicare is the subject of much ongoing debate and analysis. Medicare was designed as a program that would be funded in large part through payroll deductions (Part A) and premium payments by enrollees (Part B). There was an inherent shift of short-term wealth in Medicare's design as the employed population began to pay into the program and the retired (>65 years) population began to draw benefits. The "promise" of Medicare to the employed population was that they also would be guaranteed healthcare coverage when they reached 65 years of age. However, over the intervening decades between the 1960s and the turn of the century, the demographics of the working population and the elderly population shifted. In the 1960s, the working population of baby boomers outstripped the numbers of the elderly or retired. Currently, those same baby boomers are entering their retirement years. However, over the years during which they paid into Medicare, expansion of the population of Medicare enrollees and rising healthcare costs have used up the monies that they put into the program. Adding to the diminishing of those funds was the ongoing "borrowing" from the Medicare Trust Fund by the Congress and administrations to pay for other, nonhealthcare, programs. These shifts in population, in the use of funds and in the increasing costs of healthcare

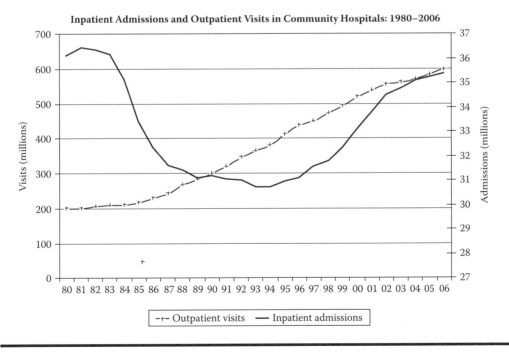

Figure 8.6   Inpatient admissions and outpatient visits in community hospitals: 1980–2006

that have outpaced overall economic growth currently drive the concern about the viability of Medicare and the need for a fundamental approach to restructuring the program.

Let us talk a bit about how the Medicare Trust Fund works. A Kaiser Foundation brief explains it well:

> Operationally, Medicare financing is managed through two trust fund accounts. The Hospital Insurance (HI) Trust Fund, into which Medicare payroll taxes and other dedicated revenue are credited, pays for inpatient hospital stays and other benefits provided under Medicare Part A. In 2006, the payroll tax provided 86 percent of all the revenue attributed to the HI Trust Fund, and 42 percent of Medicare revenue overall. The Supplementary Medical Insurance (SMI) Trust Fund is used to pay for physician visits and other Medicare Part B services as well as the Medicare Part D pre-scription drug benefit. The SMI Trust Fund is financed primarily through monthly beneficiary Part B premiums, prescription drug plan premiums, and general revenue. General revenue accounted for 76 percent of the SMI Trust Fund revenue in 2006, and 40 per-cent of all Medicare revenue, while beneficiary premiums made up 21 percent of the Trust Fund revenue and 11 percent of Medicare revenue overall. Both the HI and SMI Trust Funds are used to pay private Medicare (7).

Two major areas in which CMS has focused cost-controlling policy are (1) fraud and abuse and (2) quality of care or the effectiveness with which Medicare dollars are spent.

Regarding fraud and abuse, CMS has used the Anti-Kickback Statute, Stark I and Stark II/Self-Referral Law/Limitations on Certain Physician Referrals and the Federal Civil False Claims Act to address issues as they arise, particularly in Medicare reimbursement. A recent initiative that CMS launched was the Recovery Audit Contractor program to more aggressively seek out billing and coding errors (whether intentional or not) that cause overpayments or underpayments to providers. Under this program, auditors go into hospitals to review their billing processes and statements to determine whether or not coding of diagnosis and treatments was correct. Where errors are found, the hospital is required to compensate the Medicare program for the difference; if the error is one in which the hospital was paid too little, the Medicare pro-gram reimburses the added amount to the hospital.

Regarding quality of care, CMS has initiated programs to incentivize providers who can document certain improvements in quality processes (e.g., the pay-for-performance program) and has discontinued reimbursement for the cost of medical errors that are preventable (e.g., the "never events," such as wrong-site surgery and administration of wrong blood types, discussed in chapter 9).

8.4   Medicaid

Medicaid came into being as Title XIX of the Social Security Amendments, which were passed in 1963. Medicaid provides healthcare coverage to persons who are indigent and who are eligible for coverage based on specific criteria related to their poverty level. "Medicaid is the nation's largest publicly funded health financing program for low-income people. As a federal/state partnership, states have the option to participate or not. All states currently participate in the program. Even though Medicaid has extensive federal requirements and restrictions, states administer the program with many options. Through waivers from CMS, they have the opportunity to tailor their programs to meet their individual state medical assistance needs." (12)

In 2006, Medicaid funded approximately $320 billion of the nation's healthcare expenditure, including almost half of nursing home care. Table 8.1 depicts Medicaid expenditures by major line item for the country as a whole for 2000 through 2004.

The number of Medicaid enrollees has increased steadily since 2000. According to the CMS, there are just more than 55 million persons enrolled as of 2004. This is up from the almost 43 million who were enrolled in 2000. Of these, just more than 4 million are 65 years or older and more than 25 million are children (Table 8.2). This is important to understand in light of the statistics in Table 8.1, which indicate disparity in the proportion of Medicaid enrollees who consume a disproportionate share of the program's expenditures. That is, there are slightly over 4 million Medicaid enrollees who are 65 years or older. This is a little less than 8% of the total Medicaid enrollee population. However, persons older than 65 years consume a major portion of the nursing facility care in the United States and the total proportion of Medicaid dollars spent on nursing facility care is more than 18%. This does not account for the costs of physician visits, prescriptions, and other services used by the population older than 65 years.

Table 8.1 Medicaid Payments by Type of Service
In Millions of Dollars

	2000	2001	2002	2003	2004[1]
Total	168,443	186,914	213,491	233,206	257,722
Capitated care[2]	25,026	29,368	33,634	37,405	42,601
Clinic services	6,138	5,603	6,694	7,312	8,336
Dental services	1,413	1,897	2,309	2,595	2,867
Home health services	3,133	3,521	3,925	4,404	4,566
ICF/MR services[3]	9,376	9,701	10,681	10,861	11,141
Inpatient hospital services	24,131	25,943	29,127	31,549	34,816
Lab and X-ray services	1,292	1,623	2,157	2,365	2,699
Mental health facility services[4]	1,769	1,959	2,122	2,143	2,326
Nursing facility services	34,528	37,323	39,282	40,381	42,060
Other care[5]	14,755	16,617	19,877	21,809	24,946
Outpatient hospital services	7,082	7,496	8,471	9,252	10,196
Other practitioner services	664	762	842	882	946
PCCM services[6]	177	187	200	208	500
Prescribed drugs	19,898	23,764	28,408	33,714	39,476
Physician services	6,809	7,439	8,355	9,210	10,199
Personal support services[7]	11,629	13,135	15,363	17,245	18,497
Sterilizations	128	140	166	166	207
Unknown	496	438	1,879	1,702	1,345

Key:
1 *2004 beneficiary data is not available for Tennessee; 2003 data are represented.*
2 *HMO payments and prepaid health plans.*
3 *Intermediate care facilities for mentally retarded.*
4 *Inpatient mental health-aged and inpatient mental health-under 21.*
5 *Includes beneficiaries of, and payments for, other care not shown separately.*
6 *Primary Care Case Management Services.*
7 *Includes personal care services, rehabilitative services, physical occupational targeted case management services, speech therapies, hospice services, nurse midwife services, nurse practitioner services, private duty nursing services, and religious non-medical health care institutions.*
Source: U.S. Centers for Medicare and Medicaid Services, Medicaid Program Statistics, Medicaid Statistical Information System. (2008). Accessed October 2008. Available at: http://www.census.gov/compendia/statab/tables/08s0140.pdf

As described by the National Association of State Legislatures, "Medicaid is really three programs in one:

Table 8.2 Medicaid Beneficiaries: 2000–2004
In Thousands

	2000	*2001*	*2002*	*2003*	*2004[1]*
Total	42,887	46,164	49,755	51,971	55,078
Age 65 and over	3,730	3,812	3,886	4,041	4,289
Blind/Disabled	6,890	7,118	7,414	7,669	7,912
Children	19,018	20,340	22,369	23,992	25,639
Adults	8,671	9,769	11,238	11,679	12,303
Foster Care Children	761	775	816	839	845
Unknown	3,817	4,349	4,027	3,739	4,071
BCCA WOMEN[2]	(NA)	(NA)	5	12	19

Key:
1 2004 beneficiary data is not available for Tennessee; 2003 data are represented.
2 2Women-Breast and Cervical Cancer Assistance.

Source: U.S. Centers for Medicare and Medicaid Services, Medicaid Program Statistics, Medicaid Statistical Information System. (2008). Accessed October 2008. Available at: http://www.census.gov/compendia/statab/tables/08s0140.pdf

- a health insurance program for low-income parents (mostly mothers) and children — more than one-third of all births are covered by Medicaid;
- a long-term care program for the elderly — nearly 60 percent of nursing home residents are Medicaid beneficiaries; and
- a funding source for services to people with disabilities — paying for about one-third of the nation's bill for this population" (8).

8.4.1 Federal/State Matching Funding

Federal law provides that states may qualify for federal Medicaid matching funds only if the program is designed within specific federal requirements. These include eligibility for specific population groups, coverage for certain medical services and medical providers, and adherence to specific rules relating to payment methodologies, payment amounts, and cost sharing for Medicaid beneficiaries. States also have the authority to extend Medicaid benefits beyond the minimum federally established standards. Under these provisions, Medicaid eligibility and coverage provisions vary from state to state (8).

Two key criteria are used to derive the level of federal matching funds for which a state is eligible under Medicaid: the actual amount spent for services for enrollees that qualify as eligible for federal matching funds under Medicaid and the federal medical assistance percentage (FMAP). The FMAP is computed on the average per capita income for the state relative to the national average. By law, the FMAP cannot be less than 50%; in other words, the federal government pays at least one-half of the state's Medicaid budget. States with per capita personal incomes below the national average have received matching levels in the high 70% range. In addition to matching funds for the direct cost of care received by enrollees, states receive matching funds for the operation of their programs. Generally, this rate is set at 50%, although it may be higher under certain circumstances such as for those activities requiring skilled professionals (9).

8.4.2 Waivers

Certain programmatic requirements are placed on states in order to participate in Medicaid. These include provisions that Medicaid beneficiaries have freedom of choice of providers, that the program is offered statewide, and that services are adequately available in volume, duration, and scope to achieve their goals. Beyond this, the federal Medicaid law also allows waivers from statutory requirements so that a state can design its program to meet its unique needs or to bring innovative efficiencies to the program. The CMS may grant "program waivers" or "research and demonstration waivers." Waivers have been used, for example, in the creation of state Medicaid managed care programs (10).

8.4.3 Medicaid Managed Care

Increasingly, Medicaid programs have moved toward the use of managed care arrangements as delivery systems for Medicaid beneficiaries. Under these programs, beneficiaries may be enrolled with HMOs and managed care organizations (MCOs) or with a primary care case management system, which is a fee-for-service program that the state develops and manages. Under any of these arrangements, the beneficiary will select a specific primary care provider who is then responsible for providing and authorizing needed medical care. The patient has access to care through the primary care provider and his or her care is managed for reduced redundancy (e.g., duplication of tests) and reduced costs.

8.5   State Children's Health Insurance Program

The State Children's Health Insurance Program (SCHIP) was initiated under Title XXI of the Social Security Act as part of the Balanced Budget Act of 1997. SCHIP was designed to build on Medicaid to provide insurance coverage to "targeted low-income children" who are uninsured and not eligible for Medicaid, typically from families with incomes up to 200% of the federal poverty level or about $41,300 for a family of four in 2007. "Over the last decade, Medicaid and SCHIP together have helped to reduce the rate of low-income uninsured children by about one-third" (11).

SCHIP provides federal funds for states to expand Medicaid eligibility to children who are uninsured but who live in families with an income level above that required for enrollment in Medicaid. The program is funded with matching federal and state monies and is state administered. In 2007, the federal budgeted amount of funding for SCHIP was $5 billion.

The funding difference between Medicaid and SCHIP is that the federal match for SCHIP is at a higher percentage than it is under the Medicaid program, and children who are eligible for Medicaid are not eligible for SCHIP. This program targets children in families who live above the federal poverty-level floor but who cannot afford health insurance for their children (12). As parents have gone from welfare to work, or from job to job, and work in minimum or low-wage jobs, many are doing so without the benefit of employer-provided health insurance for their families or the ability to financially afford to pay for premiums. While many of these families support their households, their children may go without healthcare coverage due to its prohibitive cost. SCHIP provides the opportunity for them to have that coverage. This program is offered under different names in different states; for example, in Illinois, it is known as the "All Kids" program.

8.6   Other Governmentally Financed Healthcare Programs

In addition to Medicare, Medicaid, and SCHIP, the federal government provides a couple of other health insurance programs for citizens of the United States. Prominent among these are the programs offered by the Department of Veterans Affairs (VA) and the Indian Health Services (IHS).

Within the VA is the Department of Veterans Health Administration, which provides healthcare services to retired military personnel. The VA operates

174 hospitals, 696 outpatient clinics, and 250 veterans' centers throughout the country and the world (U.S. Department of Veterans Affairs, 2008). The VA is viewed as being a fully networked system, tied together with information technology that supports the input and access to medical information without geographic constraints. In 2009, the VA budget was $42.8 billion, and an increase up to $47.4 billion was established for 2010. (13)

8.6.1 Indian Health Services

The IHS is also fully funded by the federal government and provides both inpatient and outpatient services to Native Americans and Alaska Eskimos through pacts that have been in place between the U.S. federal government and the governing councils of the 553 tribes since 1787. In that year, this relationship was established and was codified in Article 1, Section 8, of the Constitution. The IHS currently provides services to approximately 1.5 million American Indians and Alaska Natives who belong to more than 557 federally recognized tribes in 35 states. (14) Figure 8.7 provides a timeline of U.S. funding of the IHS from 1975 to 2006 and reflects increasing expenditures, and Figure 8.8 provides a map depicting the locations of the IHS hospitals and other medical services.

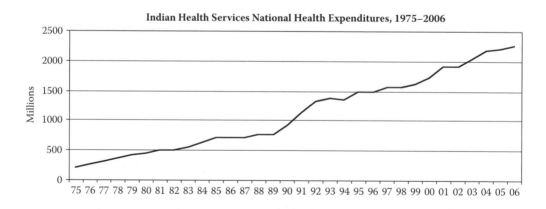

Figure 8.7   Indian Health Services national health expenditures, 1975–2006. Source: Health and Human Services, Centers for Medicare and Medicaid Services, 2008. "National Health Expenditures by types of service and source of funds." Accessed October 2008. Available at: http://www.cms.hhs.gov/NationalHealthExpendData/02_ NationalHealthAccountsHistorical.asp

8.7 The Private Sector in Healthcare Financing

We have been discussing the public sector's role and scope in healthcare financing. Governmental agencies represent about 45% of the funding of healthcare expenditures in the United States. Over 50% of overall financing comes from private sources, including employer-sponsored and paid healthcare coverage, out-of-pocket payments by individuals, and individual health insurance premiums (Figure 8.9). The dilemma that emerges in these numbers is the disproportionate share of healthcare expenditures that are made through government-based programs. Two-thirds of the nonelderly (<65 years) population have private healthcare coverage, and they account for just over 50% of healthcare expenditures. On the other hand, government sector healthcare coverage covers about 28% of the population and accounts for approximately 45% of expenditures. In dollar terms, these private sources are responsible for about $1,205,500,000 of the total cost of healthcare in the United States.

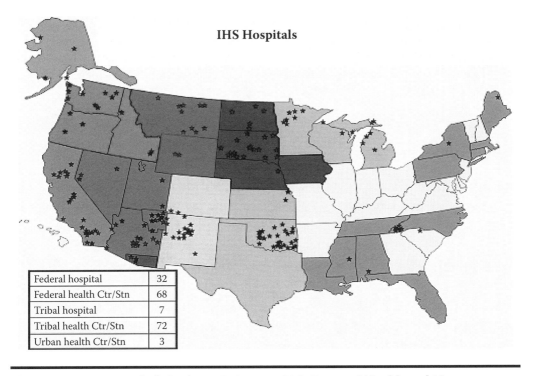

IHS Hospitals

Federal hospital	32
Federal health Ctr/Stn	68
Tribal hospital	7
Tribal health Ctr/Stn	72
Urban health Ctr/Stn	3

Figure 8.8 IHS Hospitals in the U.S. Source: U.S. Dept. of Health and Human Services (IHS). 2008. Accessed October 2008. Available at http://www.ihs.gov/ NonMedicalPrograms/chs/index.cfm?module=chs_program_directory.

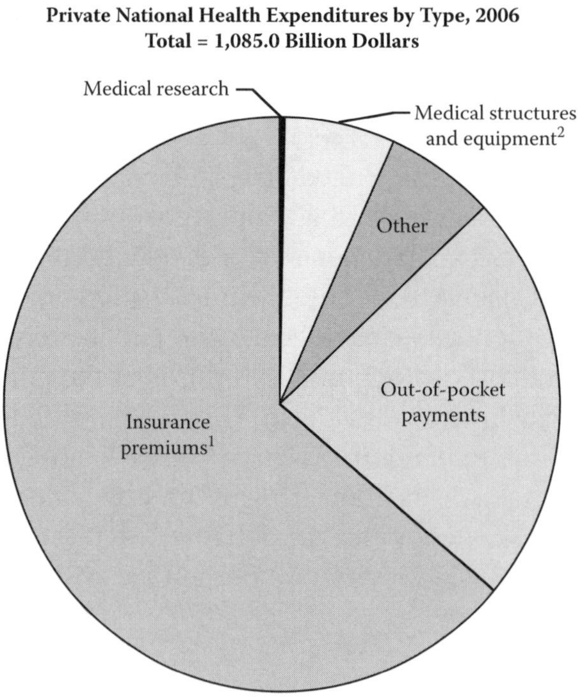

Private National Health Expenditures by Type, 2006
Total = 1,085.0 Billion Dollars

Figure 8.9   Private national health expenditures by type: 2006. Source: http://www. cms.hhs.gov/NationalHealthExpendData/02_NationalHealthAccountsHistorical. asp#TopOfPageSource

8.7.1 Employer Plans

The opportunity for employer-sponsored health insurance found its origins in a couple of initiatives that were evolving among employers in the United States in the first decades of the twentieth century. In Chicago, Montgomery Ward offered a new insurance policy to its employees in 1912. The program was primarily a life insurance policy, but it also included health and disability benefits.

While this was a beginning, the major thrust in the implementation of health insurance occurred in Dallas in 1929 when the superintendent of schools, Justin Ford Kimball, was hired by Baylor University as vice president in charge of the Baylor University College of Medicine School of Nursing. In an initiative to bolster the financial performance of the university hospital, he created a program for the Dallas teachers in which each paid $.50 a month to fund hospital care for any of them should they need it. This plan was designed as a prepaid health plan, and its success quickly spread across the country. Other provider organizations began to organize prepaid plans in a similar program. Sharing a common purpose, they all used a blue cross as the insignia or "brand," and this "symbol, in turn, led to a common name" — Blue Cross (15).

Employers started financing healthcare through employee benefit premiums in the World War II era. In a time of workforce shortages, of an economy that was booming with war production, and with inflation driven by demand and shortages, the federal government placed a moratorium on wage increases in order to control the otherwise inevitable rampant inflation. Thus, employers were not permitted to offer higher wages in order to attract or retain the employees. In an effort to keep the best and the most effective workers, employers decided to offer another financially attractive benefit to their employees. They turned to health insurance and began to offer each employee a package of health insurance benefits, thus giving employees the peace of mind that they and their families would be taken care of in the event of injury or illness. Because the federal government supported this strategy through tax breaks, employers could include the cost of health insurance as a business expense for tax purposes and thus lower their taxes. Under the same principle, taxes were not imposed on employees for the value of their new benefit. Consequently, they gained added benefit but did not see a reduction in pay. While this tax treatment of both employee and employer continues today, there is currently ongoing discussion of removing this tax benefit as one strategy to reduce the cost of healthcare and to increase the responsibility of the individual to cover more of the cost. (By way of contrast, the United Kingdom faced the same looming shortages and workforce demand as did the United States in the World War II era. The solution to the problem in the United Kingdom took the form of employers giving cars to employees, a practice that survives to the current day albeit in a more limited scope.)

Employer coverage was transformed with the expansion of managed care in the 1990s. What previously was offered to employees was indemnity plans under which employers purchase commercial health insurance for their employees and placed no focus on what was being paid to providers (the bills were sent to the insurer and, without question, were paid). As employers realized the increasing portion of their revenue that was being spent on health insurance, they turned to managed care companies to negotiate with providers for discounted rates and superimposed a care management function on services provided to covered employees and their family members. For a few years, the rate of increase in the cost of healthcare insurance plateaued, but rising employee unrest at having a limited choice of providers drove employers to expand the provisions in their coverage for employees. For example, point of service plans were developed (see p. 144).With that expansion, costs of healthcare returned to their pace of higher rates of increase.

Today, employer coverage continues to morph as employers look for more effective ways of reducing the burden of healthcare coverage on their bottom lines. Plans that engage the employee more extensively in paying for coverage and that offer incentives for employees are being implemented (e.g., health savings accounts and health reimbursement arrangements). In each of these strategies, employers attempt to place more responsibility on the employee to make careful and cost-conscious decisions in medical care. "The rationale is that if patients perceive that they are using their own funds rather than the insurer's, they will become more judicious in using those funds" (65). Employers are also designing wellness programs to reduce the cost of healthcare coverage — programs such as smoking cessation, weight loss, and exercise. Employees participating in these programs are typically offered financial incentives for achieving agreed-upon goals.

As increased responsibility is placed on the consumer in these plans that have come to be known as "consumer-directed health plans," the consumer pays higher out-of-pocket costs. A growing number of U.S. employers are designing and implementing consumer-driven healthcare plans in the form of high deductible health plans that are tied to health savings acounts (HSAs). In these plans, the employer pays into the HSA amounts that equal or approximate the high deductible. Any dollars remaining in the HSA after heatlhcare costs are paid, belong to the employee. In other words, the employee is incentivized to make good healthcare decisions.As was noted from speakers at the Healthcare Financial Management Association's Annual National Institute in 2007: "Unquestionably, consumer-directed healthcare is becoming more prevalent. And surprisingly, there was little disagreement in this group about why: employer cost-shifting" (17). Employers are looking for ways to both get their employees to take more responsibility for the healthcare costs they incur in their choices and shift some of the costs of coverage off their corporate books and onto employees.

8.7.2 Managed Care Organizations

Managed care is a system in which the insurance company influences what healthcare services patients consume, and from whom, in an attempt to manage and coordinate the patients' care and thereby limit costs. Under most managed care programs, patients have less freedom of choice in selecting providers. The original mission of managed care was to ensure that patients received wellness care and health information and had access to a variety of health resources to enable self-care. In the past few years, however, this distinction has gone away for many MCOs as they focused almost exclusively on cost control. Patient dissatisfaction with managed care plans often involves difficulty of access and a limited choice of providers who are largely motivated to deliver high-volume, low-cost care.

Some of the cost control mechanisms used by MCOs include choice restriction, gatekeeping, case management, utilization review, and practice profiling.

- ■ Choice restriction — the limitation that is put on the member in choice of providers. Typically, managed care plans contract with a network of providers, and in that contract, both parties agree to a discounted rate for the services that the provider offers. By limiting the number of providers in the network, the managed care plan can offer more business to the provider, in exchange for which the provider is willing to reduce his or her fees.
- ■ Gatekeeping — a term that was used in the early days of the growth of managed care. It is still used in some situations, but clinicians tend to view it as a misnomer for their role. The concept is that a primary care physician is the central person through whom a patient/member has access to other providers or specialists. In certain arrangements, such as many HMOs, the patient can only get to a specialist through a primary care or "gatekeeper" referral. The premises of this concept are that costs can be reduced, that the patient is cared for appropriately at the primary care level rather than at the specialist level, and that all care that can be adequately provided in a primary care setting should be done there.
- ■ Case management — the needs and values of the patient are determined, and the case manager then connects clients with appropriate providers and resources throughout the continuum of health and human services and care settings. A key role of the case manager is ensuring that the care provided is safe, effective, client-centered, timely, efficient, and equitable.
- ■ Utilization review — a mechanism through which provider and physician practice patterns are assessed; it is used to control costs. In performing a utilization review, the managed care company, or the hospital itself, considers the diagnosis on which a patient is admitted for care, continuously analyzes the reasons for which the patient is hospitalized, and anticipates a projected date or release of the patient from the hospital.

■ Practice profiling — a practice in which a physician's patterns of care are measured and assessed with the objective of impacting the clinical decision making of the physician, by, for example, encouraging the use of generic prescribing, reduction on testing, and overall reduction of costs. "Physician profiling is a method of cost control that focuses on patterns of care instead of on specific clinical decisions" (18).

There are a number of structures under which managed care companies are organized. Common types of MCOs are:

■ HMO — a comprehensive healthcare financing and delivery organization (i.e., insurer and provider of care) that provides or arranges for the provision of healthcare services to enrollees within a geographical area through a panel of providers, including hospitals, ambulatory centers, and other venues of care. Typical models within an HMO include staff models and group models. A staff model HMO provides medical care through salaried physician employees. The group model HMO delivers care through a contract with one or more medical group practices. Both of these models typically function under a capitated arrangement, meaning they are paid established rates for cases rather than billing for individual services rendered. MCOs can also be operated under an independent practice association, in which a panel of physician providers contract as a group for their services.
■ Preferred provider organization (PPO) — offers a variety of health plans that are accountable to purchasers for cost, quality, access, and other services. Hospitals, physicians, and ancillary providers may be part of a PPO. The PPO negotiates discounts with providers to make their services available to PPO members. A PPO is a combination of a fee-for-service plan and an HMO.
■ Point of service (POS) plan — allows members to choose how services are delivered at the time they are needed; it gives them the choice of going outside an approved network of providers to seek care. POS provisions may be included in HMO, PPO, or fee-for-service plans. Under them, if a member seeks care outside the network, the payer will cover the cost of that service, albeit at a lower level than the cost of a network provider. The member is then required to pay a higher portion of the cost, which he or she is often willing to do in order to see the provider of choice. POS plans developed during the low-employment economy of the 1990s, when labor was scarce and

employees resisted the limitations that many of their employer-covered plans placed on them relative to choice of providers. POS plans expanded the members' range of choice of providers.

HMOs are designed on the concepts of capitation, case management, and the provider network. Under capitation, HMOs are paid a fixed fee each month for each member of the HMO plan. This form of payment is called "per member, per month" or "pmpm," and under this arrangement, the provider is required to provide the plan participant (also known as "enrollee" in public payment plans and as "insured" in private payment plans) with all the medical care needed. The participant, on the other hand, agrees to accept a limited panel of providers from whom to seek medical care. The HMO contracts with a limited panel of providers (doctors, hospitals, etc.) at negotiated and discounted fees to provide care to plan participants. The emphasis in the HMO structure is on primary and preventive care, and these services are typically provided to the plan participant with no deductible or coinsurance, or a minimal deductible. To the plan participant, the lower cost is an enticement to accept the limitations in choice of care providers.

Key to the success of the HMO is case management, an arrangement in which a nurse or any other trained clinician follows the patient to ensure compliance with treatment regimens. It is this compliance that has been found, in many cases, to prevent the escalation of a medical condition to acute episodes.

8.8   Fee for Service

A fee-for-service insurance plan pays fees to providers for services rendered. As with most insurance, the insurance plan pays part of the expense, and the patient pays the remainder in the form of a deductible or copayment. While this plan offers freedom of choice for patients, it is usually more expensive as the focus of payment is on services rendered rather than on quality outcomes at a low cost.

8.9   Proposals for Reform of Healthcare Coverage

In the United States, the public is barraged from time to time with possible public policy proposals that would change and restructure the way in which healthcare coverage is paid. Those initiatives range from placing increased responsibility on the consumer to pay out of pocket, the cost of his or her family's medical care, to a single-payer system, to a national health insurance program, to a national health system, or to a "socialist" system."

It is important to understand several distinctions, particularly as the country debates and discusses options to create a single-payer system or a national health insurance program.

■ Public payer programs are those that are funded primarily through taxation. Primary among these are Medicare, Medicaid, the VA, and the IHS.

■ Private payer programs are those that are funded through nongovernmental sources either as employer or individual payments. With the increasing burden for healthcare payment being transferred directly to the consumer, this element of the private sources of funding is gaining increased attention as a major source of revenue for provider organizations.

■ National health insurance programs are those in which a federal level of government provides for payment of medical care for all eligible citizens. The medical providers in national health insurance systems are organized under private auspices and/or local governments. In the United States, Medicare and Medicaid are examples of national health insurance programs in that they provide coverage for specific portions of the population, in this instance, large portions of the U.S. population. National health insurance programs may be funded through a variety of arrangements, including private/public arrangement in which an employer or consumer provides a portion of funding, regional or local government funding, and/or federal funding. In the United States, national health insurance models are found in some states that have enacted mandatory health insurance for all residents. In these instances, funding is sourced from a combination of public financing through taxation, private employer coverage, and plans that allow for premiums based on sliding fee schedules. Examples of national health insurance programs are those in Germany and Belgium where both taxation and employer contributions fund a program that is administered by an arm of the federal government.

■ Socialized medicine programs are those in which either taxation or compulsory contributions fund a national insurance fund. This fund is administered by the government, and the government specifies what services will be covered. In the United States, the term "socialized medicine" is often used as a pejorative for national health insurance or a single-payer system of financing.

■ "Single payer" is a term used to describe a type of financing system. It refers to one entity acting as administrator, or "payer." In the case of healthcare, a single-payer system might be set up such that one entity — a government-run organization — would collect all healthcare fees and pay out all healthcare costs. In a single-payer system, all hospitals, doctors, and other healthcare providers would bill one entity or (more likely) a regional administrator for their services" (19).

8.10 Summary

The financing of healthcare in the United States involves a complicated mix of public and private payers and of a wide array of payment arrangements, discounted fees, patient financial responsibility, and lack of financial coverage for medical services. Over the past decade, the rate of increase in healthcare costs had been indomitable — strategies and legislative initiatives have not conquered that rate of increase. It now consumes 16% of the U.S. GDP and is expected to consume 20% in the next decade. Current approaches of consumer-directed health plans shift more of the cost to the patient. While this has been shown to have some effect on consumer behavior in use of medical services, it has also had an effect of placing greater financial burden on hospitals that find a burgeoning bad-debt account in their general ledger. While more patients are covered under SCHIP, more patients are left without coverage as employers cut back their coverage or simply do not offer health insurance. Understanding the basics of the various approaches to financing healthcare that are at play in the United States is key to understanding how the healthcare provider functions and how priorities get established.

References

1. National Coalition on Health Care. Accessed November 15, 2008. Available at: http://www.nchc.org/facts/cost.shtml
2. C. DeNavas-Walt, B. D. Proctor, and J. Smith, 2007. *Income, Poverty, and Health Insurance Coverage in the United States: 2006*. U.S. Census Bureau: Washington, DC.
3. The Henry J. Kaiser Family Foundation, 2008. "State Health Facts 2008. Total Number of Medicare Beneficiaries, 2008." Accessed December 2008. Available at: http://www.statehealthfacts.org/comparemaptable.jsp?ind=290&cat=6

4. R. Mayes, 2006. "The origins, development and passage of Medicare's revolutionary prospective payment system." *Journal of the History of Medicine and Allied Health Sciences*, 62(1), 21.

5. American Hospital Directory, 2008. "Medicare Prospective Payment System." Accessed January 2009. Available at: http://www.ahd.com/pps.html

6. Centers for Medicare and Medicaid Services, U.S. Department of Health and Human Services, 2008. "Prospective Payment Systems — General Information." Accessed December 2008. Available at: http://www.cms.hhs.gov/ProspMedicareFeeSvcPmtGen/

7. L. Potetz, 2008. "Financing Medicare: An Issue Brief. The Henry J. Kaiser Family Foundation." Accessed December 2008. Available at: http://www.cms.hhs.gov/ProspMedicareFeeSvcPmtGen/

8. National Conference of State Legislatures, 2009. "Medicaid." Accessed January 2009. Available at: http://www.ncsl.org/programs/health/h-medicaid.htm

9. Health Resources and Services Administration, U.S. Department of Health and Human Services, 2008. "Opportunities to Use Medicaid in Support of Access to Health Care Services." Accessed December 2008. Available at: http://www.hrsa.gov/medicaidprimer/

10. S. Schneider, 1997. "Medicaid Section 1115 waivers: Shifting health care reform to the states." *The State of American Federalism, 1996–1997*, 27(2), 89–109. Available at: http://www.jstor.org/stable/3330639?seq=1

11. The Kaiser Commission on Medicaid and the Uninsured, 2007. "SCHIP Reauthorization: Key Questions in the Debate — A Description of New Administrative Guidance and the House and Senate Proposals." Available at: http://www.kff.org/medicaid/upload/7675.pdf

12. Centers for Medicare and Medicaid Services, U.S. Department of Health and Human Services, 2008. "Medicaid Program — General Information. Accessed December 2008." Available at: http://www.cms.hhs.gov/MedicaidGenInfo/03_TechnicalSummary.asp#TopOfPage

13. U.S. Department of Veterans Affairs 2009. Accessed March 2009. Available at http://www.va.gov/budget/summary/2010/Fast_Facts_VA_Budget_Highlights.pdf.

14. U.S. Department of Health and Human Services, Indian Health Services, 2008. Accessed October 2008. Available at: http://www.ihs.gov/NonMedicalPrograms/chs/index.cfm?module=chs_program_directory

15. J. Asplund, February 23, 1998. "Birth of the blues." *AHA News*, 8.

16. G. R. Wilensky, 2006. "Consumer-directed health plans: Early evidence and potential impact on hospitals." *Health Affairs*, 25(1), 174–185.

17. P. Betbeze, 2007. "Straight Talk about Bad Debt." Accessed April 2008. Available at: http://www.healthleadersmedia.com/print/cfm?content_id=200202&parent=770

18. H. G. Welch, M. E. Miller, and W. P. Welch, 1994. "Physician profiling — An analysis of inpatient practice patterns in Florida and Oregon." *New England Journal of Medicine*, 330(9), 607–612.

19. Physicians for a National Health Program, 2008. "What is a Single Payer?" Accessed December 2008. Available at: http://www.pnhp.org/facts/what_is_single_payer.php

Chapter 9

Quality

9.1 Introduction

In 1999, the Institute of Medicine (IOM) released a study entitled *To Err is Human* that, for the first time, reported credible evidence of tens of thousands of deaths in hospitals that were caused by preventable medical errors — errors in drug and IV dosage; in medication administration; by wrong-site surgery (e.g., performing a surgical procedure on the patient's right knee when the left knee needed the surgery); by equipment malfunction; and by hospital-induced infections from improper, or ignored, processes for hand washing, handling of catheters, and from labeling errors. Before the report, we in healthcare knew, but were reticent to acknowledge, the outcomes of the errors that we were noting anecdotally in patient charts — available studies were not credible to us or sufficiently attention-getting to support the idea of patient deaths resulting from poor processes or from failure to follow those processes or even from lack of technology to measure the results of errors and/or of failed processes. But the IOM's report seared into our minds the startling news — as many as 98,000 people were dying in our hospitals each year as a result of preventable errors. This does not count the number of patients who were injured or who experienced an error but did not have an adverse outcome. The numbers get higher when we expand the analysis of results to include these latter adverse events that did not lead to death. To define the term "adverse event," turn again to the IOM, according to which it "is an injury resulting from a medical intervention, or in other words, it is not due to the underlying condition of the patient" (1).

The cost of medical errors is high. From 2004 to 2006, the cost of patient safety incidents was $8.8 billion, and of the 270,491 deaths resulting from errors, 238,337 were preventable (2).

After two decades of implementing a successive range of initiatives to improve quality, such as CQI, TQM, and so on, providers found themselves entering the twenty-first century face to face with a reality: people are dying while receiving medical care whose mission is life.

In this chapter, we address some of the major initiatives that have been undertaken to improve quality and prevent medical errors. We will see that the focus is on measurement, standardization, new process development, implementation of information and clinical technologies, and the design of new operational policies and, of course, education and evaluation.

9.2 Defining Quality

Quality, as beauty, may be in the eye of the beholder. Certainly, in health-care, quality is defined differently by the different players: patients, clinicians, administrators, payers (including government), and employers. Patients, as repeated studies report (3), view quality as related to the quality of the interpersonal interaction with the clinicians involved in their care and the environment of that care. When asked, they will often refer to the way in which the doctor talked to them, whether or not they feel that their situation got the attention it should get, the cleanliness of the clinical surroundings, and so on. Increasingly, as patients access more information, their perspective expands to include improved outcomes. Physicians find their definition of quality in the outcomes of their care — did the patient get well? Did the procedure go correctly? They are scientists and want to know that their knowledge and skill resolved the medical issue with which they were presented. Administrators view quality in part through the lens of the patient (i.e., through patient surveys) and in part through financial and operational data that indicate whether they are meeting their financial and volume goals. Payers have tended to measure quality based on costs. Those providers who are of lower cost have tended to be viewed as the higher quality providers. More recently, payers also include certain quality measures — particularly the process of care measures (e.g., did the heart attack patient in the emergency department get an aspirin?). They know that these types of process measures are correlated with overall improved outcomes and reduced costs of care or outlays of the premium dollars that they receive from employers and patients. Employers, who pay the premiums on health insurance benefits for employees, perceive quality in the productivity of their workforce: Was the employee given the correct medical care in a timely way? What were the costs? Was the employee back at work and productive as soon as possible?

9.3 What Is the Problem with Healthcare Quality? The IOM Reports

The IOM's report, *To Err is Human: Building a Safer Health System*, not only confirmed the number of deaths from preventable medical errors but also called for a concerted focus on improving processes. It advises that while adverse events may occur in the medical delivery setting, some of them may not be preventable, but many of them are preventable. Approximately 80% of those errors occur because of problems in the systems and processes of care. According to the Institute for Healthcare Improvement (IHI), "good people simply working harder will be insufficient to overcome the complexities inherent in today's systems of care to prevent errors and harm to patients. Errors will occur, the key is to design the care delivery systems so that harm does not reach the patient" (4).

It reported that the "increased hospital costs alone of preventable adverse drug events (ADEs) affecting inpatients are about $2 billion for the nation as a whole" (1). The report acknowledges that while the major force for reducing medical errors is the "intrinsic motivation of healthcare providers," it is also shaped by the "interaction of factors in the external and internal environment." Such factors include (1) the availability of knowledge and tools to reduce errors and measure results, (2) leadership, (3) financing mechanisms, (4) public policy initiatives, (5) organizational culture, (6) effective patient safety programs, (7) payer involvement, and (8) the will to change. In its report, the IOM laid out recommendations for addressing the problem based on a four-tiered approach, including (1):

■ establishing a national focus to create leadership, research, tools and protocols to enhance the knowledge about safety;
■ identifying and learning from errors through immediate and strong mandatory reporting efforts (and creating an environment that

encourages organizations to identify errors, evaluate causes, and take appropriate actions to improve future performance);

■ raising the standards and expectations for improvements in safety through the actions of oversight organizations, group purchasers, and professional groups;

■ creating safety systems inside healthcare organizations through the implementation of safe practices at the delivery level.

One of the core issues of efforts to improve patient safety in hospitals is the provider's reluctance to report errors due to the threat of litigation. While the IOM report acknowledges that events resulting in harm to the patient should not be kept from the public eye, the "legal discoverability of information may undercut motivations to detect and analyze errors" (1); such data should be ensured protection so that errors will not continue to be hidden. Instead, reporting of errors will provide the information to understand their root causes and to improve processes and organizational structures to prevent similar errors in the future. Some states have already enacted legislation to provide just this protection. One of them is Florida, where each healthcare facility is required to designate an appropriately trained person to inform each patient, or an individual identified under the provisions of the law, about adverse medical incidents that result in serious harm to the patient. According to the law, that notification to the patient does not constitute an acknowledgment or admission of liability and may not be introduced as evidence in court (Fla. Stat. Title 29, § 395. 1051) (5).

In 2001, subsequent to the issuance of the 1999 IOM report on safety, the IOM published a second report, *Crossing the Quality Chasm*, in which it laid out principles to guide healthcare providers in their quest to improve quality of care. *Crossing the Quality Chasm* focused on how the "health system can be reinvented to foster innovation and improve the delivery of care" (6) and presented a strategy and plan for the future. This report offered six aims for healthcare, suggesting that care delivery be:

■ safe
■ effective
■ patient centered
■ timely
■ efficient
■ equitable

The report also offered ten rules for redesign of the care delivery system:

■ Care is based on continuous healing relationships — patients should receive care when they need it and in the form in which they need it.
■ Care is customized according to patient needs and values — common types of patient needs should be met, and the system should be responsive to patient needs and choices.
■ The patient is the source of control — patients should have the information they need and [be] given the opportunity to exercise as much control as they want to take.
■ Knowledge is shared and information flows freely — patients should have complete access to their medical information and communication between patients and clinicians should be effective.
■ Decision-making is evidence based — that is, reliant on the best available scientific knowledge.
■ Safety is a system priority.
■ Transparency is necessary — the system should make available to patients and their families the information they need to make informed choices.
■ Needs are anticipated — the system should not wait to react but should anticipate patient needs.
■ Waste is continuously decreased — resources and patient time should not be wasted.
■ Cooperation among clinicians is a priority — clinicians and provider organizations should collaborate and cooperate in patient care (6).

Finally, *Crossing the Quality Chasm* addressed the environment in which patient safety would be advanced. It identified four main areas in which change is needed: application of scientific evidence to decision making; availability and use of information systems; alignment of payment policies with quality improvement; and preparing the workforce (6).

9.4 The Challenge of Quality and Safety in Healthcare Delivery

A number of factors make improvements in healthcare quality challenging. Healthcare is delivered locally, and as such, the delivery system has grown with more than 5,000 hospitals that generally operate independently of one another, with over 16,000 nursing homes that operate similarly, and with ambulatory facilities, specialty hospitals, and clinicians also functioning generally without a central focus of control (i.e., control of quality similar to that which might be found for instance in a Toyota factory). Not only is healthcare a fragmented "system," it also has as its "product" the health of very complicated human bodies mended through the complex and sophisticated structures of care delivery.

There is extensive geographic variation in the way in which care is delivered, in the clinical procedures that are used, and in the lack of evidence to support decision making across the array of possible diagnoses and clinical interventions. This variation is found not only in care delivery but also in quality and in costs that are incurred in various regions across the country. In the *Dartmouth Atlas of Health Care*, Dr. Jack Wennberg reported that "hospitals that treat patients more intensively and spent more Medicare dollars did not get better results. Similarly, the regions with the best quality and outcomes used fewer resources relative to their high-cost counterparts. Patients in low-cost, high-quality regions such as Salt Lake City, Utah, Rochester, Minnesota, and Portland, Oregon, are admitted less frequently to hospitals, spend less time in intensive care units and see fewer specialists." In other words, higher cost does not implicitly mean better quality. In many regions of the country, there is substantially more money spent while quality is poorer than in other lower cost areas (7).

9.5 Standardization/Accreditation

A first step in reducing costly variation in cost and quality may be through improved protocols of care (i.e., standardization). Standardization among hospitals and in medical education has a long history. A brief discussion of this is in order because standards organizations have been in place for decades and knowledge of what they do, and do not do, is helpful to understanding why there are so many deaths from medical errors. How does that happen when a hospital's accreditation should be a testimony to the quality of care? How does that happen when physicians must complete a rigorous course of education and licensure?

9.5.1 The Joint Commission

Although the American College of Surgeons initiated its work toward standardization in hospitals in 1913, it was not until 1951 that an accrediting body was formally founded. The Joint Commission on Accreditation of Hospitals (JCAH) was founded through the collaboration of the American College of Surgeons, the American College of Physicians, the American Hospital Association, the American Medical Association, and the Canadian Medical Association. The JCAH began offering voluntary accreditation to hospitals in 1953. A few years later, the Canadian Medical Association pulled out of the JCAH; in 1979, the American Dental Association joined as a corporate member.

Twelve years after the founding of this joint commission, when the Social Security Amendments of 1965 were passed into law, Congress provided that hospitals accredited by JCAH would be "deemed" to be in compliance with most of the Medicare Conditions of Participation for Hospitals and thus able to participate in the Medicare and Medicaid programs for reimbursement of services. This was a key incentive that drove hospitals to seek accreditation. In 1988, JCAH changed its name to the *Joint Commission on Accreditation of Healthcare Organizations* to "reflect the expanded array of accreditation programs that then included hospices and long term care, ambulatory care, home care, managed care, and behavioral healthcare programs. Program expansions in subsequent years included those for clinical laboratories, critical access hospitals, and a broad spectrum of disease-specific care and other certification programs" and brought about a further name change to simply the *Joint Commission* (8).

The Joint Commission evaluates and accredits more than 15,000 healthcare organizations and programs in the United States and provides accreditation globally in other countries under the organizational structure of Joint Commission International. It functions as an independent, not-for-profit organization. To earn and maintain accreditation and receive the Joint Commission's Gold Seal of Approval™, an organization must undergo an on-site survey by a survey team at least every three years. (Laboratories must be surveyed every two years.)

In its governance structure, a 29-member board of commissioners that includes physicians, administrators, nurses, employers, a labor representative, health plan leaders, quality experts, ethicists, a consumer advocate, and educators is appointed. Operationally, it employs approximately 1,000 people in its surveyor force and has its central office in Oakbrook Terrace, Illinois, and at a satellite office in Washington, DC. In addition to the types of organizations accredited by the Joint Commission (listed in Table 9.1), awards of Disease-Specific Care Certification are given to health plans, disease management service companies, hospitals, and other care delivery settings that provide disease management and chronic care services.

Table 9.1 The Joint Commission's Accreditation and Certification Services

Accreditation and certification services

• General, psychiatric, children's and rehabilitation hospitals

• Critical access hospitals

• Medical equipment services, hospice services, and other home care organizations

• Nursing homes and other long-term care facilities

• Behavioral health care organizations, addiction services

• Rehabilitation centers, group practices, office-based surgeries, and other ambulatory care providers

• Independent or freestanding laboratories

Finally, the Joint Commission offers a healthcare staffing services certification program (9).

9.5.2 DNV

DNV is a newly approved hospital accrediting organization. Based in Houston, Texas, its parent organization is Det Norske Ventas, a nongovernmental foundation based in Oslo, Norway. DNV bases its approach to hospital accreditation on International Organization for Standardization standards and principles. DNV was given "deemed" status by the Centers for Medicare and Medicaid Services (CMS) in 2008, which means that accreditation by it meets the criteria for Medicare conditions of participation (i.e., the hospital can participate in Medicare for reimbursement purposes) (10).

9.5.3 The National Committee for Quality Assurance

While the Joint Commission was the sole major accrediting organization in healthcare for almost 40 years, the expansion of managed care in the late 1980s and the rapidly growing interest of major employers in managed care generated an interest in a method of reviewing and reporting the level of quality with which managed care organizations operated and formally accrediting them relative to quality standards. "Back in 1989, the managed care industry was exploding onto the national health care scene. There were about six hundred managed care plans, two thirds of them not even 5 years old, with varying levels of quality and ability to assess and improve themselves" (11). In light of this growth, the Robert Wood Johnson Foundation provided grant funding to an industry trade group to assess the feasibility of creating an accrediting program that would review and evaluate managed care programs based on quality indicators.

Emerging from that study in 1990, the National Committee for Quality Assurance (NCQA) was formed as a private, 501(c)(3) not-for-profit organization. Its role is to improve healthcare quality. The key measurement and reporting tool developed and used by the NCQA continues to be the Healthcare Effectiveness Data and Information Set (HEDIS), which is now used by more than 90% of America's health plans (i.e., managed care payers) to measure performance on important dimensions of care and service (12).

NCQA health plan accreditation is designed to help employers and consumers distinguish between health plans based on quality. Health plan accreditation evaluates not only the core systems and processes that make up a health plan but also the actual results that the plan achieves on key dimensions of care and service. The review process consists of onsite and offsite evaluations conducted by survey teams of physicians and managed care experts. The Review Oversight Committee, a national oversight committee of physicians, analyzes the teams' findings and assigns an accreditation status based on a plan's compliance with NCQA standards and its performance, relative to other plans, on selected Healthcare Effectiveness Data and Information Set performance measures, such as immunization and mammography rates and member satisfaction. Developed with the input and support of employers, unions, health plans, and consumers, the NCQA sets its standards with a view to encourage health plans to continuously enhance quality (12).

9.6 Quality Improvement Initiatives

Quality improvement has not only been targeted by accrediting bodies and their efforts at standardization and measurement but also the focus of individual hospitals, governmental initiatives, and the voluntary work of other organizations and initiatives. Let us address a few of those here.

9.6.1 National Organizations and Agencies on Quality

9.6.1.1 The National Quality Forum

In 1998, a presidential commission recommended the creation of a national forum in which all of healthcare's stakeholders could come together to find ways to improve the quality and safety of healthcare in the United States. This recommendation led to the 1999 creation of the National Quality Forum (NQF), a private, not-for-profit, public benefit corporation. Its mission was and is to standardize healthcare quality measurement and reporting. The NQF has endorsed more than 400 consensus standards, including performance measures, quality indicators, preferred practices, and reporting guidelines (13).

The NQF defines its role as bringing a common approach to measuring healthcare quality and "fostering system-wide capacity for quality improvement...." While the NQF has endorsed about 400 performance measures and practices, many more are in the "measure pipeline," some in the early stages of development and others moving through the NQF endorsement process (14).

While the NQF has successfully brought together a wide array of stakeholders in developing consensus standards, there are still major challenges to quality improvement in healthcare. The NQF specifically identifies problem areas in (15)

- Error rates. Inadequate diagnosis and treatment cause unnecessary mortality and morbidity, increasing the burden, complications, and cost of treatment.
- Overtreatment. Millions of patients receive treatments each year that they do not need, leading to complications, reduced productivity, and significantly higher costs. Experts estimate that approximately 20% to 30% of health care treatments are unnecessary. Overuse has been well documented for numerous types of invasive surgery and tests; an estimated 16% of hysterectomies and 17% of coronary angiograms performed each year are unnecessary.
- Undertreatment. Studies consistently show the failure to provide effective treatments, ranging from life-saving interventions that can reduce mortality, such as taking aspirin to lower the risk of heart attack, to vaccinations that prevent serious illness in the elderly and children. Only an estimated 50% of patients receive recommended preventive care. Among individuals suffering from depression, 59% are not treated and 19% receive ineffective treatment, leading to an estimated $12 billion annual loss in employee productivity. (15)

9.6.1.2   Centers for Medicare and Medicaid Services

The CMS has a number of initiatives under way and agencies engaged in various aspects of quality standards development, measurement, reporting, and supporting quality improvement programs throughout the country. The CMS has a particular interest in ensuring that Medicare dollars are being spent effectively. Among its initiatives, the CMS has launched programs such as the Recovery Audit Contractors program under the requirements of Section 302 of the Tax Relief and Health Care Act of 2006. This program sends auditors into hospitals and other provider sites to review billing to Medicare and payments received from Medicare. When the auditor finds that the hospital has been overpaid due to billing errors, the hospital is required to reimburse to Medicare the excess funds paid; in the opposite situation, if the hospital was not paid correctly, Medicare reimburses the hospital. According to the CMS, the Recovery Audit Contractors program has provided a "mechanism for detecting improper payments made in the past, and has also given CMS a valuable new tool for preventing future payments" (16). To date, it has recovered approximately $1.03 billion (17).

The CMS has also launched other initiatives to assure quality in the care provided to Medicare beneficiaries. A few of them are discussed here.

9.6.1.3   Quality Improvement Organizations

Quality improvement organizations (QIOs) are established under the requirements of Sections 1152–1154 of the Social Security Act. In meeting this requirement, the CMS contracts with one organization in each state and the District of Columbia, Puerto Rico, and the U.S. Virgin Islands to serve as the QIO for that respective area. The selected organization then serves as that state or jurisdiction's QIO contractor. QIOs are private, mostly not-for-profit organizations, staffed primarily by doctors and other clinical healthcare professionals who perform peer review of the medical care that is provided in the jurisdiction — typically through the review of medical records, through acceptance of reports, and by responding to the inquiries and complaints of Medicare beneficiaries. The role of QIOs is to improve the effectiveness, efficiency, economy, and quality of services delivered to Medicare beneficiaries by focusing on (16)

- Improving the quality of care for Medicare beneficiaries
- Protecting the integrity of the Medicare Trust Fund by ensuring that Medicare pays only for services and goods that are reasonable and necessary and that are provided in the most appropriate setting
- Protecting Medicare beneficiaries by expeditiously addressing individual complaints

9.6.1.4   Premier Hospital Quality Incentive Demonstration

One of many quality initiatives of the CMS is the Premier Hospital Quality Incentive Demonstration. The demonstration's goal is to improve the quality of inpatient care for Medicare beneficiaries by giving financial incentives to almost 300 hospitals for measurable quality performance on certain indicators. Under this demonstration, the CMS is collecting data from these hospitals on 34 quality measures relating to five clinical conditions. Subsequently, hospital-specific performance will be publicly reported on the CMS website. Hospitals that score in the top 10% for a given set of quality measures will receive a 2% bonus payment for services to Medicare patients on top of the standard DRG payment. Hospitals that score in the next highest 10% will receive a 1% bonus. Those hospitals that do not meet a predetermined threshold score on quality measures will be subject to reductions in payment in the third year of the demonstration to further incentivize improvement. The Premier Hospital Quality Incentive Demonstration project is essentially designed to determine if economic incentives provided to hospitals are effective at improving the quality of inpatient care (18).

9.6.1.5   "Hospital Compare" Public Reporting of Performance Measures

The CMS maintains a consumer-oriented website that provides information on how well specific hospitals provide recommended care to their patients. On this site, the consumer can see the recommended care that an adult should get if being treated for a heart attack, heart failure, or pneumonia or if having surgery. The site can be accessed at http://www.cms.hhs.gov by inputting "Hospital Compare" into the search engine. At this site, the consumer can find performance data on the hospital(s) of their choice and will see how those hospitals compare with national averages and with other hospitals in a given region.

9.6.1.6   Never Events

"Never events" are, quite literally, those events that should never occur in the delivery of medical care. For example, wrong-site surgery in which the surgical procedure is performed on the left knee instead of the right knee is considered a never event. The services to correct the error and care for any adverse outcomes can cost tens of thousands of dollars or more, as well as pain and suffering for the patient. Historically, hospitals and physicians involved in performing a procedure in which a never event error occurred have been reimbursed the cost of correcting that error (e.g., performing the surgery on the correct body site and providing medical services needed to correct injury caused by surgery on healthy tissue or bone). After studying these types of events for several years, the CMS announced in 2008 that it would no longer pay the costs of never events — hospitals and doctors would be compelled to correct the error, provide all needed services to the patient, and do so at their own cost. According to the CMS, "'Never events,' like surgery on the wrong body part or a mismatched blood transfusion, cause serious injury or death to beneficiaries, and result in increased cost to the Medicare Program to treat the consequence of the error" (20).

Since the CMS has adopted the policy of no longer paying for never events, it has also encouraged state Medicaid programs to follow suit. Many have done so, as have private insurance companies. Hospitals and physicians are being denied reimbursement for the costs of fixing a condition that should not have occurred. It is expected that this negative financial incentive will spur hospitals and other providers to increase the pace of process improvement in order to reduce the number of never events that occur within their walls.

As evidence of this, hospitals have been increasingly vigilant about implementing processes that prevent never events. For example, in surgical cases, the surgeon will see the patient before surgery to confirm in detail the name of the patient, the procedure that will be done, and the site on the patient on which the surgery is to be performed. This is done repeatedly by other care providers and includes the patient placing a mark on the site on his or her body on which the surgery will be performed. Before surgery, while in the surgery suite, a "timeout" is typically called before starting surgery in order for all in the room to confirm who the patient is, what procedure is to be done, and the area of the patient's body on which to perform surgery. Many providers have also adopted the Toyota principle in which any member of the team can call a timeout during surgery should he or she observe anything questionable. (See Table 9.2 for a current list of never events.)

9.6.2 The Leapfrog Group

The Leapfrog Group is a collaboration of large employers who came together initially in 1998 to discuss how they could work together to

Table 9.2 Current National Quality Forum List of "Never Events"

Surgical Events

- Surgery performed on the wrong body part
- Surgery performed on the wrong patient
- Wrong surgical procedure on a patient
- Retention of a foreign object in a patient after surgery or other procedure
- Intraoperative or immediately post-operative death in a normal health patient (defined as a Class 1 patient for purposes of the American Society of Anesthesiologists patient safety initiative

Product or Device Events

- Patient death or serious disability associated with the use of contaminated drugs, devices, or biologics provided by the healthcare facility
- Patient death or serious disability associated with the use or function of a device in patient care in which the device is used or functions other than as intended
- Patient death or serious disability associated with intravascular air embolism that occurs while being cared for in a healthcare facility

Patient Protection Events

- Infant discharged to the wrong person
- Patient death or serious disability associated with patient elopement (disappearance) for more than four hours
- Patient suicide, or attempted suicide resulting in serious disability, while being cared for in a healthcare facility

Care Management Events

- Patient death or serious disability associated with a medication error (e.g., error involving the wrong drug, wrong dose, wrong patient, wrong time, wrong rate, wrong preparation, or wrong route of administration)
- Patient death or serious disability associated with a hemolytic reaction due to the administration of ABO-incompatible blood or blood products
- Maternal death or serious disability associated with labor or delivery on a low-risk pregnancy while being cared for in a healthcare facility
- Patient death or serious disability associated with hypoglycemia, the onset of which occurs while the patient is being cared for in a healthcare facility
- Death or serious disability (kernicterus) associated with failure to identify and treat hyperbilirubinemia in neonates

- Stage 3 or 4 pressure ulcers acquired after admission to a healthcare facility
- Patient death or serious disability due to spinal manipulative therapy

Environmental Events

- Patient death or serious disability associated with an electric shock while being cared for in a healthcare facility
- Any incident in which a line designated for oxygen or other gas to be delivered to a patient contains the wrong gas or is contaminated by toxic substances
- Patient death or serious disability associated with a burn incurred from any source while being cared for in a healthcare facility
- Patient death associated with a fall while being cared for in a healthcare facility
- Patient death or serious disability associated with the use of restraints or bedrails while being cared for in a healthcare facility

Criminal Events

- Any instance of care ordered by or provided by someone impersonating a physician, nurse, pharmacist, or other licensed healthcare provider
- Abduction of a patient of any age
- Sexual assault on a patient within or on the grounds of a healthcare facility
- Death or significant injury of a patient or staff member resulting from a physical assault (i.e., battery) that occurs within or on the grounds of a healthcare facility

Source: Center for Medicare and Medicaid Services (CMS). "Eliminating Serious, Preventable, and Costly Medical Errors – Never Events". May 2006. Accessed December 2008. Available at: http://www.cms.hhs.gov/apps/media/press/release.asp?Counter=1863

improve purchasing of healthcare for their employees and how they could impact the quality and affordability of that care. The Leapfrog Group's consortium of major companies and large private and public healthcare purchasers provides benefits to more than 37 million Americans (21). Among Leapfrog's initiatives is a program to "encourage health providers to publicly report their quality and outcomes so that consumers and purchasing organizations can make informed health care choices." Leapfrog's "hallmark initiative is its Hospital Survey which was introduced in 2001. The survey assesses hospital performance based on four quality and safety practices that are proven to reduce preventable medical mistakes and are endorsed by NQF." The consumer can go to Leapfrog's website and access the hospital survey reports. (www.leapfroggroup.org)

9.6.3 The IHI and "Pursuing Perfection"

The IHI is an independent not-for-profit organization founded by Donald Berwick, MD, in 1991 and based in Cambridge, MA. IHI positions itself as a "reliable source of energy, knowledge, and support for a never-ending campaign to improve healthcare worldwide. The Institute helps accelerate change in healthcare by cultivating promising concepts for improving patient care and turning those ideas into action" (22).

Pursuing Perfection was the brain child of IHI. Funded with $26 million over 8 years, the initiative took the IOM's five essential characteristics of quality care (safe, effective, patient centered, timely, efficient, and equitable) and crafted an approach to transforming healthcare based in part on the Toyota model for redesign of processes. "It used industry methods to improve patients' health outcomes by changing the patient care processes. It insisted that hospitals' troubles were systemic and that blame for them could not be placed at the feet of workers who were burdened by a broken system. To improve outcomes, it sought to change patient care systems" (10). All eight hospitals that participated in the initiative reported substantial improvement in care delivery and outcomes as a result of the process redesign they implemented. While the effort did not reach all its goals in transforming medical delivery, it prepared the way for subsequent campaigns to reduce medical errors.

Subsequent to the initiation of Pursuing Perfection, IHI, along with key national organizational partners, launched its 100,000 Lives Campaign, an initiative to work closely with hospitals across the country to reduce medical errors that result in death and to achieve a reduction of 100,000 deaths over an 18-month period. A total of 3,100 hospitals enrolled in the campaign. It brought awareness, focus, and education to providers and spurred new efforts at improving quality of care. Out of the experience of the 100,000 Lives Campaign, IHI has undertaken an even more ambitious campaign, the "5 Million Lives Campaign," to influence the reduction in harm (whether death or pain and suffering) caused by medical errors. The 5 Million Lives Campaign is focused on the objectives and interventions listed in Table 9.3 (23).

9.7   Payer Initiatives

Insurers are also actively engaged in quality improvement initiatives. They have, for example, adopted the principles of P4P and have followed the

Table 9.3 5 Million Lives Campaign: Objectives and Interventions

Campaign Objectives

Avoid five million incidents of harm over the next 24 months;

Enroll more than 4,000 hospitals and their communities in this work;

Strengthen the campaign's national infrastructure for change and transform it into a national asset;

Raise the profile of the problem — and hospitals' proactive response — with a larger, public audience.

Interventions

Deploy Rapid Response Teams…at the first sign of patient decline

Deliver Reliable, Evidence-Based Care for Acute Myocardial Infarction…to prevent deaths from heart attack

Prevent Adverse Drug Events (ADEs)…by implementing medication reconciliation

Prevent Central Line Infections…by implementing a series of interdependent, scientifically grounded steps

Prevent Surgical Site Infections…by reliably delivering the correct perioperative antibiotics at the proper time

Prevent Ventilator-Associated Pneumonia…by implementing a series of interdependent, scientifically grounded steps

Prevent Harm from High-Alert Medications…starting with a focus on anticoagulants, sedatives, narcotics, and insulin

Reduce Surgical Complications…by reliably implementing all of the changes in care recommended by SCIP, the Surgical Care Improvement Project (www.medqic.org/scip)

Prevent Pressure Ulcers…by reliably using science-based guidelines for their prevention

Reduce Methicillin-Resistant *Staphylococcus aureus* (MRSA) infection…by reliably implementing scientifically proven infection control practices

Deliver Reliable, Evidence-Based Care for Congestive Heart Failure…to avoid readmissions

Get Boards on Board…by defining and spreading the best-known leveraged processes for hospital Boards of Directors, so that they can become far more effective in accelerating organizational progress toward safe care

Source: Institute for Healthcare Improvement (IHI), 2008. 5 Million Lives Campaign. Accessed December 2008. Available at: http://www.ihi.org

lead of Medicare in refusing to pay for "never events." They call for evidence-based interventions in patient care and incentivize physicians to use evidence-based tools when making clinical decisions. They also seek to improve patient satisfaction and financially reward providers who achieve high patient satisfaction scores.

9.8 Evidence-Based Medicine

In the 1990s, evidence-based medicine (EBM) emerged as a way to improve and evaluate patient care. In EBM, research evidence is used in conjunction with the patient's values to make decisions about the best medical care for the patient. Using EBM, individual clinical expertise is integrated with the best external evidence from research and practice. "It is the conscientious, explicit, and judicious use of current best evidence in making decisions about the care of individual patients" (24).

What clinicians know about illnesses, diseases, diagnoses, injuries, and their effective treatment is expanding continuously. However, the health professional of today cannot keep pace with the rapidly growing body of knowledge that is generated by research and the researcher's analysis of the enormous amount of data that is made available through the implementation of information systems that support the real-time collection of data from the clinical and business sectors of healthcare. In using EBM, clinicians apply their expertise and experience, expanded upon by current research literature, to provide the patient with the best advice and judgment possible in the current state of the art of medicine. Practice guidelines and clinical protocols are established using best evidence and research to help clinicians and their patients make the best decisions regarding clinical care.

9.9 The Medical Home

Chronic conditions afflict at least 45% of the U.S. population, and more than 80% of Medicare enrollees have at least one chronic condition. When there is a lack of coordination of care of these individuals and management of their conditions, costs escalate. Duplicative diagnostic tests are often ordered by different providers, patients return home from a medical visit or hospitalization without clear understanding of medication protocols, often to be readmitted within a short period, others receive medications that interfere with one another, and overall their care is not appropriately managed. The concept of the medical home was developed to address these issues. The medical home is not necessarily a place: it is a team of primary care providers (doctor, nurse, other clinicians) whose role it is to coordinate the care of the patient. They provide primary care services, but beyond that, they also (1) arrange specialist care, (2) follow up with patients to ensure that they are compliant with diet and exercise plans and that they understand which medications they are prescribed and how and when to take them, and (3) overall manage the care of the patient in order to prevent the onset of acute episodes of one or more of the chronic conditions that the patient has. Medical home initiatives are under way across the United States under the auspices of hospitals, health systems, and medical groups. Initial studies of the effectiveness of medical homes indicate that they can significantly reduce costs and can support the patient in living a more productive and healthy life (25).

9.10 Tools for Quality Improvement

9.10.1 Dashboards

A quality dashboard is a graphic array of information that highlights an organization's performance in a number of designated areas of quality. It is meant to be visual, with focused data contained in a small amount of space. "The dashboard should include [at least one] variable from each of the following nine topic areas: outcomes frequently compared with nationally established benchmarks; critical national initiatives; publicly reported data; progress on local initiatives; patient satisfaction; patient complaints and potential lawsuits; significant incidents; workforce issues, such as retention; and peer review summaries. Specifics will vary by hospital and service area, but when all variables are put together, a comprehensive picture emerge will emerge" (26).

9.10.2 Benchmarking

Benchmarking is the "process of establishing a standard of excellence and comparing a business function or activity, a product, or an enterprise as a whole with that standard. As a component of total quality management, benchmarking is a continuous process by which an organization can measure and compare its own processes with those of organizations that are leaders in a particular area."

Benchmarking must be a team process because the outcome will involve changing current practices. This will impact the entire organization. The team should represent a cross-section of the organization and include members who have subject knowledge; communications and computer proficiency; skills as facilitators and outside contacts; and, very important, sponsorship of senior management. Benchmarking requires quantitative measurement of the subject. "The process or activity that you are attempting to benchmark will determine the types of measurements used. Benchmarking metrics usually can be classified in one of four categories: productivity, quality, time and cost-related" (27).

9.11 Summary

Quality improvement is one of the most demanding and needed areas of work in healthcare. Following the 1999 release of the IOM report *To Err is Human*, healthcare providers, payers, and consumers faced the irony and horrors of tens of thousands of patients dying and many more suffering adverse events due to preventable medical errors. In the decade since the release of the IOM report, new initiatives and incentive programs have been launched from every sector of healthcare to improve patient safety, reduce errors, and restore a sense of confidence in medical delivery. The errors that occur are primarily generated not through the negligence of caregivers but through the lack of processes that can be put in place to reduce errors. Hospitals are now required to publicly report their outcomes on key indicators that indicate their accuracy in following correct protocols for care. Hospitals are ranked against one another for these indicators, and as the public becomes more aware of and accesses these rankings, it is believed they will make more informed choices about their care providers. This is only one of many steps that address the issue of quality improvement in healthcare — there are many others as discussed in this chapter. Additionally, information systems and the use of process improvement methods, such as Six Sigma and Toyota's "lean" methods, as well as payer incentives for quality improvement and disincentives related to never events, are all initiatives that hover over and drive improvement.

References

1. Institute of Medicine, 1999. *To Err is Human: Building a Safer Health System*. Executive Summary. National Academies Press: Washington, DC, pp. 4 and 6.
2. "Medical Errors Cost U.S. $8.8 Billion, Result in 238,337 Potentially Preventable Deaths, According to HealthGrades Study." Accessed December 14, 2008. Available at: http://www.healthgrades.com
3. B. Rosenthal, R. Fernadopulle, H. Song, and B. Landon, 2004. "Paying for quality: Providers' incentives for quality improvement." *Health Affairs*, 23(2), 127–141. http://content.healthaffairs.org/cgi/content/full/23/2/127
4. L. Botwinick, M. Bisognano, and C. Haraden, 2006. "Leadership Guide to Patient Safety." IHI Innovation Series white paper. Institute for Healthcare Improvement: Cambridge, MA, p. 2.
5. L. Kasprak, 2007. "OLR Research Report: Medical Error Reporting by Hospitals." Accessed December 6, 2006. Available at: http://www.cga.ct.gov/2007/rpt/2007-R-0471.htm
6. Institute of Medicine, 2002. *Crossing the Quality Chasm: A New Health System for the 21ˢᵗ Century*. National Academies Press: Washington, DC.
7. "New Study Shows Need for a Major Overhaul of How United States Manages Chronic Illness." Accessed November 2008. Available at: http://www.dartmouthatlas.org/press/2006_atlas_press_release.shtm
8. http://www.jointcommission.org/AboutUs/joint_commission_history.htm. Accessed October 15, 2008.
9. http://www.jointcommission.org/AboutUs/Fact_Sheets/joint_commission_facts.htm. Accessed October 15, 2008.
10. J. DerGurahain, 2008. "DNV setting new standard." *Modern Healthcare*. Available at: http://www.modernhealthcare.com/article/20081027/REG/810249995
11. S. L. Isaacs and D. C. Colby (Editors), 2008. *The Robert Wood Johnson Anthology: To Improve Health and Health Care. Volume XI*. Jossey-Bass: San Francisco, CA, p. 11.
12. About NCQA. Available at: http://www.ncqa.org/tabid/675/Default.aspx. Accessed October 24, 2008.
13. http://www.qualityforum.org/about/work.asp. Accessed October 24, 2008.
14. http://www.qualityforum.org/about/NPP/. Accessed October 19, 2008.
15. http://www.qualityforum.org/about/history/quality.asp. Accessed October 15, 2008.
16. http://www.cms.hhs.gov/RAC/. Accessed December 16, 2008.
17. CMS, 2008. The Medicare Recovery Audit Contractor (RAX) Program: An Evaluation of the 3-Year Demonstration, p. 15. Available at: http://www.cms.hhs.gov/RAC/Downloads/RAC%20Evaluation%20Report.pdf
18. http://www.cms.hhs.gov/qualityImprovementOrgs/. Accessed December 16, 2008)

19. CMS, 2006. "Eliminating Serious, Preventable, and Costly Medical Errors — Never Events." Available at: http://www.cms.hhs.gov/apps/media/press/release.asp?Counter=1863

20. The Leapfrog Group Fact Sheet. Available at: http://www.leapfroggroup.org/about_us/leapfrog-factsheet. Accessed December 6, 2008.

21. http://www.ihi.org/ihi/about. Accessed December 19, 2008.

22. C. J. McCannon, A. D. Hackbarth, and F. A. Griffin (2007). Miles to go: An introduction to the 5 Million Lives Campaign. *The Joint Commission Journal on Quality and Patient Safety*, 33(8), 477–484.

23. A. D. Oxman, D. L. Sackett, G. H. Guyatt, and the Evidence-Based Medicine Working Group (1993). *Users' Guide to Evidence-Based Medicine*, 270(17), 2093–2095. American Medical Association: Chicago, IL.

24. P. H. Keckley and H. R. Underwood 2007. *The Medical Home: Disruptive Innovation for a New Primary Care Model — A Report from the Deloitte Center for Health Solutions.*

25. L. Larson. "How to Drive a Quality Dashboard." Interview with Eric D. Lister, MD., managing director of Ki Associates, Portsmouth, NH.

26. H. R. Benson, 1994. An introduction to benchmarking. *Radiology Management*, 16(3), 35–392.

Chapter 10

Public Health

10.1 Introduction

Public health in the United States is the "other arm" of healthcare delivery and gathering of statistics on health-related matters including both the incidence of disease and the environment in which disease occurs. Public health services are provided through governmental support at the local community, state, and federal levels. The core roles of public health service are "assessment, policy development and quality assurance" (1). These services generally serve the needs of those less fortunate persons who otherwise lack access to medical care and of those who may be subject to infectious diseases.

Public health finds its orientation in the health of the population, looking broadly at the conditions and incidences of disease or injury that occur within the population and providing services (e.g., immunizations) and information to control the spread of disease. While the public health sector of society is a critical part of the infrastructure of providing medical care in the United States, it is not generally tied into the private sector providers of care (both nonprofit and for-profit medical providers). Public health is distinct from the providers and payers that serve the insured and the uninsured in the United States. Nonetheless, public health services are provided not only through government agencies, but also through a plethora of voluntary organizations in communities across the country such as the Red Cross, which voluntary clinics operated by faith-based and civic-minded groups in poor access areas of metropolitan and rural locations, shelters, and by neighborhood centers where health screening and basic assistance may be provided. While these are important organizations in the overall support of public health in the United States, this chapter will focus on the work provided by government agencies that are involved in research, data collection and dissemination, and the provision of primary medical services.

Public health services are offered at all levels of government. While there are responsibilities that are similar at each level (e.g., gathering and reporting of vital health data), each has duties that reflect the level of government at which they are organized. For example, the local health department may be involved in owning and operating primary care clinics, while at the state and federal levels, a corollary responsibility is to provide health services after a major disaster, e.g., post-Katrina.

10.2 Role of Public Health

The IOM defines the role of public health as "what we, as a society, do collectively to assure the conditions for people to be healthy." At one point, the work of public health agencies was focused primarily on the physical health of the population, but by the turn of the twenty-first century, that role took on a more comprehensive and holistic role. In 1994, a collaboration of stakeholders from all sectors of public health and all levels of government undertook an effort to help national, state, and local public health agencies focus on their public health goals. In this effort, they defined the vision of public health as "Healthy People in Healthy Communities," a vision that suggests that all factors that impact a population's health should be considered cohesively in order to improve health status. The collaborative defined the mission of public health to be "Promote physical and mental health and prevent disease, injury and disability." The subsequent six public health responsibilities that will support the achievement of this mission are to:

- Prevent epidemics and spread of disease
- Protect against environmental hazards
- Prevent injuries
- Promote and encourage healthy behavior
- Respond to disasters and assist communities in recovery
- Assure the quality and accessibility of health services

These responsibilities apply to all levels of public health — federal, state, county, city, and community. Each has a part in assuring, for example, that citizens are protected against environmental hazards. For instance, the local public health department will assume authority when a public building contains suspect or potentially harmful materials, will ban smoking in public places in order to prevent harm to the public from second-hand smoke, and will provide public health clinics and/or educational programs to assure that otherwise underserved populations will have access to certain basic services. At a state level, similar responsibilities will be carried out through activities such as licensure of professionals to assure the quality of health-care practitioners, provision of mental health hospitals to assure accessibility to services that would otherwise be unavailable to persons without the financial means to pay for those services, and the funding of educational programs. Likewise, the federal level of government holds responsibility in each of the six areas. For example, the Centers for Disease Control and Prevention (CDC) gathers data for assessment of epidemics and takes measures to prevent outbreaks of disease and helps to provide reporting and services in times of disaster and the Food and Drug Administration (FDA) is responsible for the safety of the food supply and of drugs. While there are other agencies at each level of government that have defined responsibilities in public health, each has interconnected roles. For example, health data are gathered on an ongoing basis — the local government collects vital statistics and reports those to the state level from which, in turn, they are reported to the federal level of government (the CDC). On a global scale, the same six responsibilities apply to public health agencies. Particularly, the World Health Organization holds leadership, oversight, and administrative responsibility in these six areas for countries around the globe. It is important to understand that from the local to the global level, public health responsibilities are inter-related through reporting mechanisms and through programs of education and planning/implementation of health services that relate to improving and maintaining the health of populations.

10.3 Public Health at the Federal Level

At the federal level, public health services are organized within the executive branch of the government, under the auspices and direction of the Department of Health and Human Services (HHS). HHS is organized with 11 operating divisions, including the Office of Public Health and Science, or OPHS, each of which has responsibility for specific health-related functions. At the state level, public health services are offered through a state department of health (named differently in different states), and at the local level, these services are offered by a city or county health department where essential functions relate to data gathering and reporting, food and environmental safety, etc., and through which clinics provide basic preventive and primary care services directly to populations in need of them.

10.3.1   Office of Public Health and Science

The OPHS is composed of 12 core public health offices and the Commissioned Corps, a uniformed service of more than 6,000 health professionals who serve within the HHS and other federal agencies and may be assigned to research institutions or other organizations.

The assistant secretary for health (ASH) serves as the primary advisor to the secretary of the U.S. HHS on matters involving the nation's public health. The ASH oversees the Office of Public Health and Science for the department (2).

HHS works closely with state and local governments, and many HHS-funded services are provided at the local level by state or county public health agencies and clinics or through private sector grantees. The department's programs are administered by 11 operating divisions, including eight agencies in the U.S. Public Health Service and three human services agencies. In addition to the services, divisions within the department enable the collection of national health and other data.

The overall HHS Budget for FY 2008 was approximately $707.7 billion. The department employs over 64,000 professionals and staff (3). The department includes more than 300 public health programs, covering a wide spectrum of activities. These include:

- Health and social science research
- Preventing disease, including immunization services
- Assuring food and drug safety
- Medicare (health insurance for elderly and disabled Americans) and Medicaid (health insurance for low-income people)
- Health information technology
- Financial assistance and services for low-income families
- Improving maternal and infant health
- Head Start (preschool education and services)

- Faith-based and community initiatives
- Preventing child abuse and domestic violence
- Substance abuse treatment and prevention
- Services for older Americans, including home-delivered meals
- Comprehensive health services for Native Americans
- Medical preparedness for emergencies, including potential terrorism

10.4 History of Public Health Service

The origins of public health are found in centuries of evolving health services and assumption by various departments of government for the protection of the health of the population. In the formative days of the country, the United States shared a common interest with countries in Europe where commercial interests and the viability and vibrancy of towns and cities were reliant upon a healthy population — one that could be productive and could contribute to the economic growth of the municipality and the country. With the growth of crowded cities along the East Coast of the United States, the vulnerability of the population to disease was endemic. Sanitary conditions were challenging, and the lack of public services to address health issues was a concern to governments and to business.

As cities took on responsibility to assure the sanitary conditions of the city and to provide medical care to their indigent residents who otherwise would not have access to care, the numbers of clinics and almshouses where physicians could work grew. However, along the coastal cities, people working on ships were not residents and fell outside the responsibility of the city. To control diseases entering the country from merchant ships, to provide services to treat the illnesses and injuries that seamen experienced, and to support the vitality of the maritime trades, the federal government put in place the Marine Hospital Service in 1798. Under the Marine Hospital Service, hospitals and clinics came into being in major coastal cities and ports. First among these was the Marine Hospital set up in Boston Harbor. As this initiative evolved over the next century, the Marine Hospital Service became the U.S. Public Health Service in 1912 and took on responsibilities that reached well beyond seamen to include the urban and rural populations across the country.

A major part of the U.S. Public Health Service is the Commissioned Corps, which was put in place by the Congress in 1889. The corps was initially designed to be a "mobile force of physicians to assist the nation in fighting disease and protecting health" (1, 362). Today, under the direction of the Surgeon General, "the U.S. Public Health Service Commissioned Corps is an elite team of more than 6,000 full-time, well-trained, highly qualified public health professionals dedicated to delivering the Nation's public health promotion and disease prevention programs and advancing public health science" (4).

It was not until the mid-nineteenth century that local governments also began to formally take on responsibility for the health of their communities. In the middle of the nineteenth century, the Report of the Sanitary Commission of Massachusetts prepared by Lemuel Shattuck, a statistician, documented the results of unsanitary and environmental conditions, and related death and disease, to the level of unsanitary conditions in which people lived (5). This report recommended that cities establish structures such as Boards of Health to oversee and have authority over infrastructure (e.g., where businesses whose products or processes impacted the environment, disposal of waste, location of cemeteries). However, it was not until almost a decade and a half later that New York took it upon itself to investigate the living environments of the city and the measures of illness and deaths in the city. The study reported such egregious unsanitary conditions that the first Board of Health was created in New York and given the authority and the resources to address the city's unsanitary conditions. This Board of Health signaled a turning point for public health in the United States as cities took on responsibility to assure the sanitary conditions of the city and to provide medical care to their indigent residents who otherwise would not have access to care. Clinics and almshouses, where physicians worked, grew as cities took on this responsibility.

10.5 U.S. Public Health Service Today

The office of the Secretary of the HHS has overall responsibility for the range of public health services that is available in the United States. While the Centers for Medicare and Medicaid Services (CMS) is situated within HHS, this department also has 11 operating divisions that have a role in the public's health. Eight of these operate under the Office of Public Health and Science (Figure 10.1). The departments within the Public Health Service are organized with the following functions:

1. The Administration for Children and Families (ACF) is "responsible for federal programs that promote the economic and social well-being of families, children, individuals, and communities." ACF's "mission is to promote the economic and social well-being of children, youth, families, and communities, focusing particular attention on vulnerable populations such as children in low-income families, refugees, Native Americans, and people with developmental disabilities. ACF administers programs carried out by state, territorial, county, city, and tribal governments as well as by private, non-profit, and community- and faith-based organizations designed to meet the needs of a diverse cross-section of society" (7).

   In FY 2009, the president's budget request of $45.6 billion for the ACF included both mandatory (preappropriated and entitlement) and discretionary programs. In 2008, the budget for ACF stood at $43.8 billion, supporting the Low Income Home Energy Assistance Program (LIHEAP), the Child Care and Development Block Grant (CCDBG) program, Head Start, and Refugee and Entrant Assistance, Temporary Assistance for Needy Families (TANF), Child Care Entitlement, Child

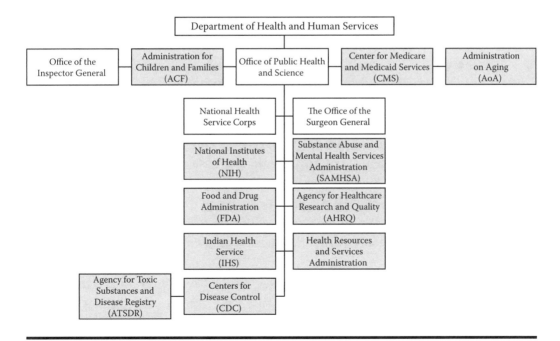

Figure 10.1.   Organization structure of U.S. Office of Public Health and Science. The 11 operating divisions are shaded in gray. Source: http://www.hhs.gov/about/orgchart/

Support Enforcement, and Foster Care and Adoption Assistance. The agency is staffed by about 1,300 full-time equivalent (FTE) positions (7).

2. Administration on Aging (AoA) is the federal agency responsible for advocating on behalf of older persons and to address their concerns. In addition to promoting the awareness of the needs and concerns of older persons among the various agencies of government, the AoA works "with and through the Aging Services Network to promote the development of a comprehensive and coordinated system of home and community-based long-term care that is responsive to the needs and preferences of older people and their family caregivers" (8).

   The AoA's FY 2009 budget request to Congress of $1.38 billion reflected a funding level approximately equal to the appropriated funding for FY 2008. That budget is targeted to strengthening the national aging services network in meeting the challenges presented by the aging of the baby boomers and the need for more options for long-term living and the agency's "commitment to support the core programs that provide home and community-based long-term care services to millions of older persons through the national aging services network. The network, made up of state, tribal, and area agencies on aging as well as more than 29,000 community-service providers, has been a proven force in advancing healthy living and independence in the community and serves over 9 million individuals each year" (8).

3. The Agency for Healthcare Research and Quality (AHRQ) supports and performs health services research initiatives that seek to improve the quality of healthcare in America. AHRQ's mission is to improve the quality, safety, efficiency, effectiveness, and cost-effectiveness of healthcare for all Americans. It carries out this work through support and funding of research initiatives carried out by and in academic institutions, hospitals, physician practices, and other healthcare provider organizations (9).

   AHRQ's FY 2009 estimate proposed budget of slightly more than $325.6 million is a decrease of $8.9 or 2.7% from the FY 2008 enacted level of funding (10).

4. The Agency for Toxic Substances and Disease Registry (ATSDR) is the nation's public health agency for chemical safety. First organized in 1985, ATSDR was created by the Comprehensive Environmental

Response, Compensation, and Liability Act (CERCLA) of 1980, more commonly known as the Superfund law. Under its CERCLA mandate, ATSDR's work falls into four functional areas:
- Protecting the public from hazardous exposures
- Increasing knowledge about toxic substances
- Educating healthcare providers and the public about toxic chemicals
- Maintaining health registries

The ASTDR is organized under the structure of the CDC. It employs about 400 people, and its FY 2009 budget proposal of $72.8 million was slightly less than the $74 million FY 2008 enacted level (11).

5. The CDC functions under its mission "to promote health and quality of life by preventing and controlling disease, injury, and disability." The agency is the "primary Federal agency for conducting and supporting public health activities in the United States. Composed of the Office of the Director, the National Institute for Occupational Safety and Health, and six Coordinating Centers/Offices, including environmental health, and injury prevention, health information services, health promotion, infectious diseases, global health and terrorism preparedness and emergency response, CDC employs more than 14,000 employees in 40 countries and in 170 occupations" (12).

   The FY 2009 president's budget submission includes a total funding level for CDC/ATSDR of slightly more than $8 billion (excluding ASTDR), reflecting a decrease of approximately $412.1 million below the FY 2008 enacted level (13).

6. The FDA is "responsible for protecting the public health by assuring the safety, efficacy, and security of human and veterinary drugs, biological products, medical devices, our nation's food supply, cosmetics, and products that emit radiation. The FDA is also responsible for advancing the public health by helping to speed innovations that make medicines and foods more effective, safer, and more affordable; and helping the public get the accurate, science-based information they need to use medicines and foods to improve their health" (14).

   The FDA "is the federal agency responsible for ensuring that foods are safe, wholesome and sanitary; human and veterinary drugs, biological products, and medical devices are safe and effective; cosmetics are safe; and electronic products that emit radiation are safe. The FDA also ensures that these products are honestly, accurately and informatively represented to the public" (15). Its more than 10,000 staff includes scientific and technical professionals and a professional staff whose goal is to protect and advance public health.

The FY 2009 president's budget request for FDA is $2.4 billion. This represents a total program level increase of $129.7 million above the FY 2008 enacted level (16).

7. The Health Research and Services Administration (HRSA) defines itself as "the nation's access agency" — improving health and saving lives by making sure the right services are available in the right places at the right time. It is the primary federal agency for improving access to healthcare services for people who are uninsured, isolated, or medically vulnerable.

   Comprising six bureaus and 12 offices, HRSA provides financial support to healthcare providers in every state and U.S. territory. Its grantees provide healthcare to uninsured people, people living with HIV/AIDS, and pregnant women, mothers, and children. They train health professionals and improve systems of care in rural communities. HRSA also oversees organ, tissue, and blood cell (bone marrow and cord blood) donation and vaccine injury compensation programs and maintains databases that protect against healthcare malpractice and health care waste, fraud, and abuse (17).

   The FY 2009 HRSA Budget request of $5.8 billion was about $1 billion below its enacted funding level for FY 2008 (17).

8. The Indian Health Service (IHS) is the agency responsible for providing federal health services to American Indians and Alaska Natives. The IHS is the principal federal health care provider and health advocate for Native Americans people and in that role currently provides, as mentioned earlier, health services to approximately 1.5 million American Indians and Alaska Natives who belong to more than 557 federally recognized tribes in 35 states (18).

   The FY 2009 budget request for the IHS was just over $3.3 billion — a decrease of $21 million below the FY 2008 enacted funding level (19).

9. The National Institutes of Health (NIH) is the primary federal agency for conducting and supporting medical research. Composed of 27

institutes and centers, the NIH provides leadership and financial support to researchers in every state and throughout the world. The NIH traces its roots to 1887 with the creation of the Laboratory of Hygiene at the Marine Hospital in Staten Island, New York. With headquarters in Bethesda, Maryland, the NIH has more than 18,000 employees.

The FY 2009 budget request for the NIH was just over $29.2 billion, equal to the FY 2008 appropriation. Included in these funds is specific funding for the Type I Diabetes Initiative, for the AIDS research program, and for the Global Fund for HIV/AIDS, Tuberculosis, and Malaria. More than "83% of the NIH's funding is awarded through almost 50,000 competitive grants to more than 325,000 researchers at over 3,000 universities, medical schools, and other research institutions in every state and around the world. About 10% of the NIH's budget supports projects conducted by nearly 6,000 scientists in its own laboratories, most of which are on the NIH campus in Bethesda, Maryland" (20).

10. The Substance Abuse and Mental Health Services Administration's (SAMHSA's) mission is one of "building resilience and facilitating recovery." Through its three centers and supporting offices, SAMHSA engages in program activities to carry out this mission. With a fiscal year 2007 budget of nearly $3.3 billion, SAMHSA funds and administers a portfolio of grant programs and contracts that support state and community efforts to expand and enhance prevention and early intervention programs and to improve the quality, availability and range of substance abuse treatment, mental health, and recovery support services — in local communities — where people can be served most effectively (21).

The FY 2009 president's budget request cut SAMHSA's budget by over 50% from its enacted level in 2008. Its 2009 budget of $15.6 million is meant to fund 21 grants and one contract continuation at a 53% reduction (22).

11. The mission of the Office of the Inspector General (OIG) is to protect the integrity of HHS programs, as well as the health and welfare of the beneficiaries of those programs. With its more than 1,500 professional staff, the OIG is responsible to report both to the secretary of HHS and to the Congress program and management problems and recommendations to correct them. The FY 2009 OIG budget request was for $46 million, which was about $3 million above its FY 2008 enacted amount (23).

10.5.1   *The Office of the Surgeon General*

The Office of the Surgeon General oversees the operations of the 6,000-member Commissioned Corps of the U.S. Public Health Service and provides support for the Surgeon General in the accomplishment of his other duties. "The Surgeon General serves as America's chief health educator by providing Americans the best scientific information available on how to improve their health and reduce the risk of illness and injury. The Surgeon General is appointed by the President of the United States with the advice and consent of the United States Senate for a 4-year term of office and reports to the Assistant Secretary for Health" (24).

10.6 Healthy People 2010

In 1979 the Surgeon General issued his report, *Healthy People,* and with it laid the foundation for a national prevention agenda. At the beginning of each decade since then, a broad-based consultation process has brought scientific knowledge to the development of national health objectives that could, and have, served as the basis for the development of state and community health prevention and intervention plans and have helped identify the measures for success in the implementation of those plans. The Healthy People initiative establishes overall objectives for the nation relative to top priority health concerns that have been enunciated through the process of consultation with leading scientists, healthcare, and community leaders and professionals from both the public and private sectors. As a group, the leading health indicators reflect the major health concerns in the United States at the beginning of the twenty-first century. These indicators were selected based on their importance as public health issues and on the basis of their ability to motivate action, the availability of data to measure progress.

The leading health indicators are:

■ physical activity
■ overweight and obesity
■ tobacco use
■ substance abuse
■ responsible sexual behavior
■ mental health

- injury and violence
- environmental quality
- immunization, and
- access to health care (25)

The Healthy People initiative and reports have helped guide the proactive public health initiatives of states, counties, and municipalities across the country. Through a process of ongoing prioritization and program implementation, each of these levels of government has been able to bring about improved health status for the groups on which they have focused resources for health improvement. From their ongoing programs, they report before and after data relative to the level of achievement they have accomplished for their particular geographic area and targeted population(s).

10.7 Summary

The role of public health is an important one in the context of healthcare delivery in the United States. Both the public and private sectors share goals and responsibilities for the health of communities and of individuals. While the public health orientation is primarily on population health and that of the healthcare delivery system is primarily focused on the individuals, each is inherently tied to the other. Populations are made up of individuals, and individuals can have substantial impact on populations (e.g., in the spread of disease). While the early history of public health and healthcare delivery systems were integrally tied together, that relationship fragmented as the private sector of healthcare delivery grew and as the growing population demanded increasing attention to health hazards and overall health status. Following major disasters in the United States (e.g., 911, Katrina, fires in California, floods in the Midwest, a bridge collapse in Minnesota) and with the threat of major acts of terrorism, it has become clear that linkages between the two sectors are critical to the health and safety of the population and of individuals. This demand is driving increased collaboration, information sharing, and information technology infrastructure to support the sharing and caring that is needed in times of crises and in the interests of improved health status of the population. Healthy People 2010 is just one initiative that reflects a wider participation in initiatives to achieve these ends.

References

1. H. A. Sultz and K. M. Young, 2009. *Health Care USA: Understanding Its Organization and Delivery*, 6th Edition. Jones and Bartlett: Sudbury, MA.
2. http://www.hhs.gov/ophs/. Accessed September 17, 2008.
3. http://www.hhs.gov/about/whatwedo.html/. Accessed July 31, 2008.
4. http://www.usphs.gov/aboutus/questions.aspx#whatis. Accessed July 31, 2008.
5. http://www.deltaomega.org/shattuck.pdf. Accessed July 29, 2008.
6. http://www.usphs.gov/aboutus/questions.aspx#whatis. Accessed July 29, 2008.
7. http://www.acf.hhs.gov/programs/olab/budget/2009/sec1_comb_ov_2009cj. pdf. Accessed August 22, 2008.
8. http://www.aoa.gov/about/org/org.aspx. Accessed July 22, 2008.
9. http://www.ahrq.gov/about/stratpln.htm. Accessed July 22, 2008.
10. http://www.ahrq.gov/about/cj2009/cjweb09a.htm#Summary. Accessed July 20, 2008.
11. http://www.cdc.gov/fmo/PDFs/FY09_ATSDR_CJ_Final.pdf. Accessed July 20, 2008.
12. http://www.cdc.gov/about/resources/facts.htm. Accessed July 1, 2008.
13. http://www.cdc.gov/fmo/PDFs/FY09_CDC_CJ_Final.pdf. Accessed July 20, 2008.
14. http://www.fda.gov/opacom/morechoices/mission.html. Accessed July 20, 2008.
15. http://www.fda.gov/comments/regs.html. Accessed July 20, 2008.
16. http://www.fda.gov/oc/oms/ofm/budget/2009/Execsum/1_Exec_Summary.pdf. Accessed July 20, 2008.
17. http://www.hrsa.gov/about/default.htm. Accessed July 22, 2008.
18. http://www.ihs.gov/PublicInfo/PublicAffairs/Welcome_Info/IHSintro.asp. Accessed July 21, 2008.
19. http://www.ihs.gov/NonMedicalPrograms/BudgetFormulation/documents/ FY%202009%20IHS%20Budget%20CJ%20Submission.pdf. Accessed July 19, 2008.
20. http://officeofbudget.od.nih.gov/ui/HomePage.htm. Accessed August 20, 2008.
21. http://www.samhsa.gov/About/background.aspx. Accessed August 20, 2008.
22. http://www.samhsa.gov/Budget/FY2009/SAMHSA_CJ2009.pdf. Accessed August 20, 2008.
23. http://www.oig.hhs.gov/organization.html. Accessed June 16, 2008.
24. http://www.surgeongeneral.gov/about/index.html. Accessed June 15, 2008.
25. http://www.healthypeople.gov. Accessed June 15, 2008.

Chapter 11

Technology
Medical and Information Technologies

11.1 Introduction

Technology is one of medicine's most fascinating dimensions. In a relatively short time, medicine has gone from a basic understanding of infection and its causes to the ability to successfully perform multiple organ transplants, to reattach limbs after they have been severed, to prolong life with procedures and drugs that were unheard of only decades ago. From an information perspective, increased volume and complexity of the information that is generated at the bedside and the need to pass that information from provider to provider, to improve the safety of patient care, to respond to the many and varied payer programs that dominate the U.S. financing of healthcare, and to improve efficiency and effectiveness in order to drive down an out-of-control rate of increase in healthcare costs have made implementation of healthcare information technology (IT) mandatory. Yet, both of these areas, advances in medical technology and deployment of IT, consume huge investments and require time and process change. In this chapter, both kinds of technologies will be briefly introduced. Both are vast fields and will require further study by the person whose professional life in healthcare management brings them into day-to-day involvement with either IT or advances in medical technology.

11.2 Medical Technology

Medical technology is comprised of the wide range of procedures, tools, and interventions that are used to diagnose and treat healthcare problems. Here we will focus on pharmaceuticals, research, pharmaceuticals, genomics, and medical devices.

11.3 Pharmaceuticals

New drugs come to market on an ongoing basis as pharmaceutical companies and researchers discover and develop new compounds to address the health conditions that affect human beings. However, the process of getting those new drugs to market is complex, time consuming, and very costly. Developing and getting a new drug to market can cost a company hundreds of millions of dollars. Because of the investment,

> Innovations in the health sciences have resulted in dramatic changes in the ability to treat disease and improve the quality of life. Expenditures on pharmaceuticals have grown faster than other major components of the health care system since the late 1990s. Consequently, the debates on rising health care costs and the development of new medical technologies have focused increasingly on the pharmaceutical industry, which is both a major participant in the health care industry and a major source of advances in health care technologies (1).

11.3.1   Clinical Trials Research

The clinical trials process from laboratory bench to the marketing shelf takes an average of 15 years for each drug. Only 20% to 25% of drugs that begin a phase I clinical trial actually succeeding to market (1). Most of the drug development process is spent in the laboratory and in human clinical trials. The last component is the Federal Drug Administration's final review and approval process (Figure 11.1).

11.3.1.1   Preclinical Research

The first step of a clinical trial is the preclinical research. This phase begins in the laboratory with teams of scientists working together to create

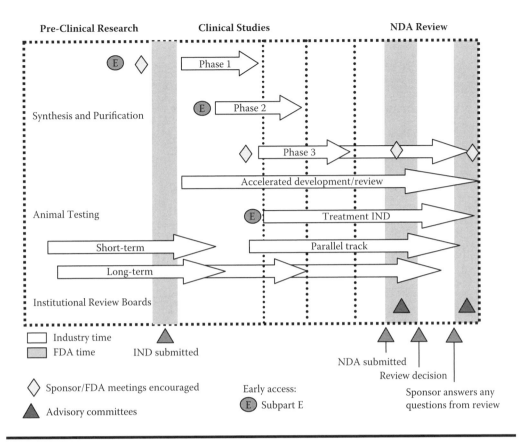

Figure 11.1 The New Drug Development Process: Steps from Test Tube to NDA Review. Source: FDA. 2009. "The New Drug Development Process: Steps from Test Tube to New Drug Application Review." Accessed January 7, 2009. Available at: http://www.fda.gov/CDER/HANDBOOK/DEVELOP.HTM

compounds that will treat a physiological condition and then ends with animal studies that evaluate how the compound works in a living organism. This phase may be completed in short-term testing of 2 weeks to 3 months or long-term testing of a few weeks to several years depending on the planned use of the substance. Once the preclinical research is complete, the drug sponsor can complete an investigational new drug application (NDA) and submit this to the Center for Drug Evaluation and Research at the FDA (21). There are about 5,000 drug compounds that are evaluated in this pre-clinical phase each year.

11.3.1.1.1 Phase I: Clinical Studies

Phase I of clinical studies involves the initial introduction of an investigational new drug into humans. These studies are typically conducted in 20 to 80 healthy volunteer subjects and are designed to determine the drug's effect on humans, including the metabolic and pharmacological actions, the side effects associated with increasing doses, and, if possible, to gain early evidence on effectiveness, and any potential early indications of the effectiveness of the drug. Phase I trials typically take from one to one and a half years to complete and cost about $10 million (2). If they do not reveal unacceptable levels of toxicity, then the drug generally moves into phase II of the clinical trials.

11.3.1.1.2 Phase II: Clinical Studies

Phase II includes the early controlled clinical studies in several hundred test subjects (people with the disease or condition that the drug targets). In these studies, the researchers seek to obtain preliminary data on the effectiveness of the drug for a particular indication or indications in patients. This phase of testing also helps determine the common short-term side effects and risks associated with the drug. Typically, phase II of the clinical trials takes about two years to complete and costs tens of millions of dollars to. About one-third of drugs introduced into phase II complete this phase successfully.

11.3.1.1.3 Phase III: Clinical Studies

In phase III, research is expanded with controlled and uncontrolled trials. The objective of this phase is to study the effectiveness, safety, and overall benefit-risk relationship of the drug. Phase III studies include several hundred to thousands of people and are performed to provide an adequate basis for extrapolating the results to the general population and transmitting that information in the physician labeling. Phase III takes about three years to complete and costs an average of $40 million. The success rate for drugs in phase III is 70% to 90% (3).

11.3.1.1.4 Phase IV: Approval process

Every new drug completes a new drug application (NDA) process prior to marketing by its sponsor company. An NDA includes all preclinical animal testing and human clinical trial data and analyses. Following phase IV trials studies may continue and are used to learn about the treatment's long-term side effects, risks, benefits, and optimal use, or to test the product in different populations of people like children (2).

11.3.2   Basic Scientific Research

The reason we do basic biomedical research lies in the fact that the living organisms especially higher organisms like human beings are highly complicated (4). It is estimated that there are about 30,000–40,000 human genes (5). Although all the human genome sequences were completed in 2003, much is left to know about the essential component of the cell "protein" and the complex network it creates, which renders cell diversity. For major diseases such as cancer, heart disease, arthritis, and diabetes, the cellular and molecular changes involved in the development of these conditions are so complicated that better understanding of the basic molecular and cellular mechanisms is necessary in the diagnosis, treatment, and prevention of these diseases. For some acute infectious diseases like smallpox and anthrax, effective treatment is possible only after the cause of disease is well characterized. Another important reason for conducting basic biomedical research is that diseases are more likely to be diagnosed and cured at an early stage if mechanisms of the diseases are thoroughly understood. Costly machinery and surgical procedures can therefore be avoided, which will save a great deal of money in the future (5).

Funding for biomedical research comes from both public and private resources. In year 2003, the National Institutes of Health (NIH) contributed about 28% of total medical research funding mostly through universities. In the private sector, pharmaceutical, biotechnology, and medical device companies contribute about 58% through their research and development departments (6). Some small amounts of research are also carried out or funded by private nonprofit foundations.

The National Institutes of Health (NIH) is part of the U.S. Department of Health and Human Services and is the primary agency of the government for biomedical research. Its goal is to expand our knowledge in medical and associated sciences to help prevent, detect, diagnose, and cure disease and disability. NIH is divided into an intramural and an extramural divsions. The former conducts research in the NIH main campus in Bethesda, Maryland, and the latter is in charge of the funding of research outside of NIH. In 2006, NIH invested 83% of its $28 billion funding to extramural research, which supports 200,000 researchers in 3,000 institutions nationwide. Unlike private companies, NIH focuses more on basic research other than applied research. In 2007, 56.1% of the funding was invested in basic research and technology development versus 40.8% in applied research (7).

11.3.3 Genomics

The Institute of Medicine (IOM) in 2005 defined genomics research as "An emerging field that assesses the impact of genes and their interaction with behavior, diet and the environment on the population's health." A human genome includes all the genetic material (DNA) of an organism.

Having access to the human genome sequence is a powerful tool in understanding the pathogenesis of disease. The ability to identify candidate genes, hypothesize about their function by identifying the family of genes to which they belong, and identify the same or similar genes in other organisms that permit experimentation has greatly accelerated the pace of research. As dramatic as these advances have been, however, far more remains to be learned about how genes affect human health. The field of pharmacogenomics is poised for this study.

Pharmacogenomics is the study of how an individual's genetic inheritance affects the body's response to drugs. This field holds the promise of personalized healthcare (PHC) in which drugs of the future might be tailor-made for individuals and thereby adapted to each person's own genetic makeup. Environment, diet, age, lifestyle, and state of health can all influence a person's response to medicines, but understanding an individual's genetic makeup is thought to be the key to creating personalized drugs with greater efficacy and safety. Pharmacogenomics is expected to make possible a future of

- More powerful medicines
- Better, safer drugs the first time they are given to a patient
- More accurate methods of determining appropriate drug dosages
- Advanced screening for disease
- Better vaccines
- Improvements in the drug discovery and approval process
- Decrease in the overall cost of healthcare (8)

Genomics and PHC also must be discussed from the perspective of the ethical issues they raise relative to confidentiality and potential discrimination by insurers and employer. The Genetic Information Nondiscrimination Act, also known as GINA, was signed into law in 2008 and is intended to protect Americans against discrimination in health insurance and employment and to pave the way for people to take full advantage of the promise of personalized medicine without fear of discrimination (9).

IT will play a critical role in realizing the potential of PHC, because information (data) and knowledge management are at its core. PHC has the potential to transform the quality, safety, and value of healthcare. The disease areas that will see early adoption of PHC solutions include diseases with both genetic and environmental causes, including autism, heart disease, diabetes, obesity, and cancers. The technological advances that will enable PHC include the electronic medical record (EMR), mobile medical devices and monitors, storage technology improvements, and high-performance computing technologies. IT technologies and security at provider and payer organizations will have to change to accommodate PHC and data requirements and address privacy concerns. PHC has the potential to improve the return on healthcare investment, but the evidence is still sparse (10).

The healthcare and pharmaceutical industries have never before been faced with greater pressure—both internal and external—to speed drug production and move toward PHC. Meanwhile, new discoveries in genomics and the widespread use of high-throughput research technologies are producing massive amounts of data to enable the better understanding of disease. In addition, healthcare providers are being pushed to capture patient data electronically. These forces all contribute to researchers' and medical providers' increasing need to leverage information assets and align the clinical and research environments in order to identify and understand the underlying mechanisms of disease for the transformation of healthcare (4).

11.4 Information Technology

11.4.1   Introduction

Information is central to medicine and medical care delivery. Without accurate and complete information, the incredible opportunities that are in medicine's future, the quality of care, and the comprehensiveness of care cannot be realized. Yet, this huge industry that is healthcare remains the last bastion in the implementation of the information systems and information sharing. Healthcare provider organizations lag far behind other sectors of the U.S. economy in the implementation of electronic information systems.

While we can go to any ATM in the world and perform banking functions with our "back home" bank, we cannot go from one provider to another and have access to our health information in order to interact with that provider. In most cases, we find ourselves repeating the same information for input into the paper records of the new provider or into a stand-alone computer system, and that provider cannot immediately electronically access the results of any tests or interventions we might have had previously.

We wait while the fax machine, or even the postal service, delivers our information in hard copy to the new provider's office.

In that scenario, not only must we as patients wonder about the adequacy of the information that is accessed by hard copy but we must also be concerned that our providers are hamstrung by the lack of timely and complete information that would make them more efficient and productive — and would reduce the costs of healthcare. In the digital age, the lack of electronic health information will not work.

Beyond the issue of what we and our providers face is the financial impact of lack of electronic access to our medical records. This lack leaves us open and subject to duplicate testing, prescription errors, burdensome administrative requirements, inefficiencies, and other costly consequences. As our healthcare costs consume over 16% of our GDP and continue to rise at alarming rates while the quality of our outcomes puts us further and further behind those in other developed countries, the imperative for the fully functional, shared electronic health record (EHR) grows.

As stated by the American Hospital Association (AHA): "Research has shown that certain kinds of technology (IT) — such as computerized physician order entry (CPOE) computerized decision support systems, and bar coding for medication administration — can limit errors and improve care by ensuring that the right information is available in the right place at the right time to treat patients" (11).

11.5 Why the EHR?

Increasingly, the call for the EHR is being heard from all sectors of society — employers, consumers, government, researchers, payers, and healthcare organizations.

■ *Employers* want to assure that the money they are spending on healthcare supports the productivity of a healthy workforce. Rising healthcare costs are compelling employers to transfer more of that cost onto their employees. They want to see more information sharing, reduction in errors, and greater efficiency in healthcare. The electronic sharing of data is key to getting beyond the paper record and the administrative burden that it incurs and reducing costly errors and duplication of services.

■ *Consumers* want information, and as they reach deeper into their own pockets, they seek out the information that will help them make better choices. 80% of Americans, or about 113 million adults, have searched for information on at least one of seventeen health topics according to a report from the 2006 PEW Internet and American Life Project (13).

■ *Government*, at both the federal and state levels, is calling for the implementation of EHRs across the country. States are funding the development of health information exchanges and the Center for Medicare and Medicaid Services (CMS) has several initiatives underway to foster the development and implementation of EMRs. Among these initiatives is the Pay-for-Performance (P4P) program, which financially rewards providers for documented improved performance and quality — documentation which is highly reliant on the availability of the electronic record. Recently, CMS announced a plan to reward physicians who write electronic prescriptions with a 2% bonus in 2009. This bonus would diminish over the next several years, until by 2013, those physicians who are not using electronic prescribing will be penalized 2%. Outside of these incentives to encourage the adoption of electronic records, other federal government initiatives from the Agency for Health Research and Quality (AHRQ) and other agencies provide grants to communities to support the implementation of electronic records for the maintenance and sharing of clinical data. Current AHRQ initiatives include a 10-year strategy to provide more than $260 million in grants and contracts in 41 states to support and stimulate investment in healthcare IT (14). Additionally, the legislature, in its ongoing efforts to find ways to address rising healthcare costs, is considering increasingly strong legislative proposals for the implementation of the EHR.

■ While the availability of the EHRs offers the opportunity for more data than has ever been available before, the provisions for privacy and confidentiality in the handling of those data have created challenges to *researchers* to accessing that data. Researchers have expressed frustration in the implementation of HIPAA provisions that impede their ability to access clinical data from patient records.

■ *Payers* have for a long time been among the prime movers for the EHR. The EHR supports the transfer of data, thereby reducing the administrative workforce needed to handle paper; it supports the accuracy of data and billing statements; and, above all, it supports the reduction in duplication of testing that drives up healthcare costs. Payers can be a "winner" in the financial benefits of the electronic implementations by reducing payments to providers for duplicate testing and for errors in billing.

■ Finally, *healthcare organizations* need to deploy EMRs. Since the release of the 1999 IOM report *To Err is Human* gave us credible evidence that some 98,000 people have been dying in hospitals each year as a result of preventable medical errors, hospitals have been under the cloud of poor performance based on the startling data in this report. Major investments have been, and are being, made, to correct those errors. Systems that support computerized provider order entry (CPOE) and medication management offer the opportunity to establish new processes to improve the accuracy of ordering, filling, and administering drugs, IVs, and IV additives and, ultimately, of reduction in errors. Electronic systems also are essential to supporting the accurate transfer of medical record information when patients are transitioned from one care provider to another (e.g., from emergency room, to surgery, to ICU, to acute care unit..

■ The Rand Corporation has estimated that implementing clinical and administrative health information systems will generate cost savings of $162 billion annually (15). This will come about as a result of reduction of duplication of laboratory and radiology tests and of administrative work (16.). Paper administrative costs can be as high as $0.20 per dollar of costs.

However, implementation of the EHR is challenging for providers. They are making hundreds of millions of dollars of investments in IT, yet many have not yet seen a measurable financial return on investment (ROI) on those dollars. Additionally, they face the need for fundamental change in processes of care, a change that means that the behavior of clinicians must change in order to achieve adoption of the new systems. Physicians and hospitals tend to resist sharing their patient information, however, and in order for the EHR to live up to its definition, all clinicians need to participate in providing access to that information.

Importantly, the implementation and use of the EMR has proven to be central to improving the safety, efficiency, and effectiveness of medical care. Chapter 9 discussed the scope and impact of medical errors and the number of deaths that occur in hospitals due to preventable medical errors. These errors arise from hand-written orders for drugs that cannot be deciphered; from errors that occur in the transition of patient care from one provider to the next; of errors in patient identification in treatment or medication administration; of miscommunicated clinical information; and other process points. In order to fix the processes that are open to error, the electronic record is critical.

11.6 EMR or EHR: Which Is It?

There has been a tendency to use the terms *electronic medical record*, or *EMR*, and *electronic health record*, or *EHR*, interchangeably. However, the industry has generated distinct definitions of the two, and it is useful to understand this distinction.

Healthcare Information and Management Systems Society (HIMSS) defines the EHR as "a longitudinal electronic record of patient health information... that spans across the continuum of care, generated by one or more encounters in any care delivery setting. Included in this information are patient demographics, progress notes, problems, medications, vital signs, past medical history, immunizations, laboratory data and radiology reports. The EHR has the ability to generate a complete record of a clinical patient encounter — as well as supporting other care-related activities directly or indirectly via interface — including evidence-based decision support, quality management, and outcomes reporting" (17).

In other words, the EHR supports the sharing of information among providers regardless of their organizational affiliation or geographic location. With it, hospitals can access the information that physicians record and that are in the records of other hospitals; patients do not need to provide basic personal and insurance information in each different provider's office. Those providers can simply retrieve that information from the EHR.

The EMR, on the other hand, provides for the recording of all patient information in the hospital or physician office that has adopted the EMR. While that hospital or provider may be completely paperless, the EMR does not support the sharing of that data with other providers of care. So, the EMR might be considered a "subset" of the EHR — it becomes an EHR when there is full access to the data by other providers and by the patient.

11.7 Components of the EHR

HIMSS Analytics has developed a model of EHR adoption that identifies the components of an EHR and that suggests the seven-stage progression by which those components are typically adopted by healthcare providers.

In the model (Table 11.1), the EHR is identified as being fully implemented only when the organization has adopted and begun using the various components. For example, at stage 1 of adoption, the provider has its laboratory, radiology, and pharmacy departments computerized. As it moves to stage 2, it will adopt a central data repository (CDR), a common medical vocabulary (CMV), a clinical decision support system inference engine (CDSS), and possibly, document imaging. In stage 3, clinical documentation is implemented, the CDSS performs error checking and notification, and the radiology department's picture archiving and communication system (PACS) is available for access outside of the department. Stage 4 requires that computerized practitioner order entry (CPOE) is implemented for clinicians to electronically record orders for tests, procedures, and medications. These orders are then accessed by the department that will be responsible for carrying them out and by other clinicians and staff who need to know of the order. At stage 4 the functionality of the CDSS includes clinical protocols that provide the clinician point-of-care information about adopted processes for care for the diagnosis and condition of the patient. In stage 5, closed loop medication administration is implemented affording the entire medication

Table 11.1 EMR (SEHR) Adoption Model, 2006

		% of U.S. Hospitals		
		Final	3rd Qtr	1st Qtr
Stage 7	Medical record fully electronic; CDO able to contribute to ICEHR as byproduct of SHEMR	0.0%	0.0%	0.0%
Stage 6	Physician documentation (structured templates), full CDSS (variance & compliance), full PACS	0.1%	0.1%	0.1%
Stage 5	Closed loop medication administration	0.5%	0.5%	0.6%
Stage 4	CPOE, CDSS (clinical protocols)	3.0%	2.7%	2.5%
Stage 3	Clinical documentation (flow sheets), CDSS (error checking), PACS available outside Radiology	18.0%	14.2%	11.2%
Stage 2	CDR, CMV, CDSS inference engine, may have Document Imaging	38.8%	42.9%	46.7%
Stage 1	Ancillaries – Lab, Rad, Pharmacy	18.9%	21.8%	19.8%
Stage 0	All Three Ancillaries Not Installed	20.7%	17.9%	19.0%

Source: Healthcare Information and Management Systems Society, HIMSS Analytics. 2007. "Essential of the US Hospital IT Market 2007." Accessed October 12, 2008. Available at: http://www.himssanalytics.org/docs/e07_chapterintro.pdf

administration process, from placement of the order to administration of the medication to the patient, to be electronically managed. As the provider achieves stage 6, physician documentation will be fully functional, and a full CDSS and the radiology PACS will be implemented. Only at stage 7 is the full EHR recognized. At this point, the patient record is fully electronic (the EMR) and that record is accessible on a shared basis with other providers, even those outside the organization (18).

11.8 Health Information Exchange (HIE)

Health information exchange refers to the technology and process infrastructure that supports the sharing of clinical and other patient data within a geographic region and among the organizationally unrelated providers of care in that region. As individual healthcare provider organizations develop and implement the EMR, there is another initiative under way in defined geographic regions to develop the technical and governance infrastructure to support sharing of data throughout the region. Many states are funding these initiatives, and federal dollars are flowing into them. The ultimate objective of these initiatives is to create the capability and environment through which a National Health Information Network can be developed to support the sharing of health information among providers and patients nationwide and, particularly, in the event of a disaster such as Hurricane Katrina.

The 2008 eHealth Initiative Annual Survey of Health information Exchange at the National, State, and Local Levels revealed that a number of HIEs are already reporting that they are in the advanced stage or operational stage of HIE development. Operational HIEs have grown considerably in the past few years: in 2006 there were 26; in 2007 there were 32; and in 2008, 42 reported that they were operational. There is increasing "momentum for the use of health information exchange to improve the quality, safety, and efficiency of healthcare in the U.S." (18).

The two major challenges that HIEs face are stakeholder commitment and of finding an effective business model that can support a sustainable enterprise. In gaining stakeholder commitment, the HIE needs not just the support but also the cooperation and participation by providers in the region. If those providers see the sharing of information as a competitive threat or if they have concern about the privacy of the information, they will resist active participation and financial support for the HIE. The second challenge is that of building a viable business model. In order to succeed, the HIE requires that providers who access data through the electronic network pay a fee for that access or provide another form of financial support. If providers do not see competitive advantage in accessing information through the HIE, they will resist making the financial commitment.

11.9 The Personal Health Record

The personal health record (PHR) can be viewed as a component of the EHR or as the electronic record that is fully in the control of the patient, i.e., it is that person's individual record and as such data can be entered into it by the patient, and it can be accessed by the patient at any point. Sharing of that information is under the control of the patient who can give providers access as they choose to do so. The Markle Foundation's Connecting for Health collaborative has defined the PHR as an electronic application "that enables individuals or their authorized representatives to control personal health information, supports them in managing their health and well-being and enhances their interactions with health care professionals" (20).

A number of employers have made the PHR available to their employees as a part of their health plan in order to encourage the employee to take charge of their healthcare and to assure consistent and complete information not only about their medical care but also about their wellness activities (exercise, alternative healthcare, and so on). Microsoft and Google have introduced PHRs and made them available to their customers to use.

A key ingredient of the PHR will be the ability to integrate or interface it with the EMR, and how the PHRs will impact medical discussion and decisions at the point of care. The PHR will drive an awareness and understanding among providers of the concept of patient-centered care: the model in which the patient is fully engaged in decision-making and decisions involve, at their core, the needs, values, and input of the patient.

11.10 Types of Information Systems in Healthcare

The healthcare IT environment consists of three major components: application software, hardware, and network connectivity. It also requires information systems in two major domains: the administrative or business functions of healthcare and clinical functions. Healthcare software must support the many varied functions in each of these two domains, and it must serve to integrate information between both domains. In order to have a fully functioning EHR, the systems must support full sharing of information, on a need-to-know basis, among clinicians, administrators, patients, and others involved in care regardless of their geographic location or the venue of care (hospital, physicians office, rehabilitation, ambulatory center, etc.)

Now we may question, why is that a problem? We can, for example, use our ATM card at almost any ATM location around the world — not only from different banks, but in different countries. The difference is that the transaction-based world of ATMs is much less complex in technological design than the healthcare environment. While healthcare requires transactional systems, it also requires systems that support point-of-care decision making, which occurs when the clinician is seeing the patient and ordering tests, providing medication, or performing other clinical functions. They require data warehouses that not only store data but have the capacity to support evidence-based medicine by making clinical research and findings available at the clinician's fingertips, so that he or she has immediate access to the latest research findings and to best practices.

The challenges in making this happen are plentiful. First of all, unless an organization designs and builds its own system, those systems are generally designed and developed by a variety of vendors leading to interoperability issues. While standards organizations are working continuously on the development of standards, there is still not one set of standards to support the full integration of information systems. The challenge of implementing systems as interoperable elements of a whole is daunting. Not only do legacy or older existing information systems not comply with standards, but currently available systems are, for the most part, not available from one source that will have designed them to function interoperably.

Table 11.2 lists the major areas in which information systems are used in healthcare provider organizations. The major categories of healthcare IT systems as listed in the table are clinical systems and administrative systems. Clinical systems serve in the patient care settings such as at the bedside, in the surgical suite, the emergency department, the laboratory, radiology, pharmacy the doctor's office, and so on. Administrative systems, on the other hand, support the business and management functions of the organization — such areas as billing, accounts payable, reporting, human resources, supplies management, and so on. Historically, U.S. hospitals have been focused on IT systems that support financial or business functions and scheduling functions — such as billing, accounts payable, accounts receivable, physician scheduling, and so on. Not only are these two domains the major focus of integrated information systems, but other functions in

Table 11.2   Healthcare IT Domains

Healthcare IT Applications

Clinical Systems

Patient Administration Systems:

- Point-of-care systems
- Case management applications
- Disease management applications
- Emergency department applications
- Critical care systems
- Surgery systems
- CPOE (Computerized Practitioner Order Entry)
- Ambulatory information systems

Ancillary Clinical Systems:

- Order entry systems
- Medical imaging
- Radiology systems
  - Medical imaging systems
  - Radiology Information System
  - PACS (Picture archiving and communication systems)
- Pharmacy information systems
- Laboratory information systems
- Ambulatory information systems

Administrative Systems

Financial Management Systems
Billing Systems
Scheduling Systems
Productivity Systems
Decision Support System (DSS)

healthcare also need to be supported. Consider such activities as research and education, which are highly reliant on the data that information systems can make available. The bottom line is that the design, development, and implementation of fully integrated information systems for healthcare providers are as complex as the organizations themselves.

11.11 Challenges to IT Adoption

IT adoption is critical to healthcare's future, and its development is continuing with major investments of time, money, and resources going into both organizational systems and into health information exchanges. There are, however, major challenges on this path to achieving the ubiquitous EHR. These challenges include

- Cost: Healthcare annually invests less than 2% of its revenue in information systems. Very recently, CMS announced that it anticipates spending close to $300 billion on IT within the next five years. In an environment of continuously rising healthcare costs, tightening reimbursement systems, and other investment priorities (e.g., buildings, medical technologies, nursing education programs) to address the problems plaguing healthcare, it can be anticipated that information systems professionals will feel greater and greater pressure to justify the investment that is required to get to a viable information infrastructure.

- Process change/adoption: It has been demonstrated repeatedly that when information systems are implemented without attention to the process change that is inherent in the implementation, and without attention to the need for processes to drive the IT decisions rather than vice versa, the investment that is made in IT is ineffectual and often leads to the abandonment of the entire IT system. Process change implies behavior change, and this is one of the more difficult elements to change in an organization. The investment in IT does not stop at the purchase or development of the software; the organization must be prepared to make investments in understanding its processes, in changing those processes, and most importantly in patiently but assertively educating its clinicians and other professional and support staff to change the way in which they work and to accept change in the interrelationships that are central to the work of the organization.

- Interoperability — standards development: Information exchange is key to improving quality, reducing costs, and achieving more efficiency and effectiveness in healthcare delivery. Key to information exchange is the development of IT standards and use of those standards in the development of information systems, and key to standards development is achieving consensus among the many standards development organizations (SDOs), and their constituents that cover the field of healthcare IT standards. Achieving consensus continues, but at a slower pace than the pace of investments that are being made in healthcare IT. As the National Institute of Standards and Technology puts it:

The healthcare industry has many standards development organizations (SDOs) developing specifications and standards to support healthcare informatics, information exchange, systems integration, and a wide spectrum of healthcare applications. The large number of healthcare organizations and standards that exist, or are in-development, make it difficult to monitor and track the overall landscape of healthcare standards. In-turn, this impedes standards coordination and harmonization efforts among SDOs, and frustrates efforts by users and organizations to identify, understand, adopt, and deploy needed standards (23).

A number of SDOs (see Table 11.3) are actively engaged in standards development. This is occurring in four areas of healthcare IT. As described in Table 11.3, they include content standards, structure standards, messaging standards, and functional standards.

Standards development in healthcare faces a number of challenges including:

■ Legacy systems: These are information systems that a hospital or health system has had in place for any number of years and that the organization continues to rely on for certain functionalities, such as billing, accounts receivable in business systems and laboratory, radiology, and other clinical departments. The significance of the issue of legacy systems is that they were typically built without regard for their interoperability or ability to integrate with other systems acquired later. As the provider organization moves to implement systems with enterprise-wide functionality (e.g., the EHR), that organization faces the challenge of integrating the older system with the new and of integrating clinical systems to develop the fully functional EHR.

■ Security and privacy: Security of information is critical both to the organization and to the patient. Under HIPAA, healthcare organizations engaged in the electronic transfer of data (e.g., billing to payers) are required to have systems in place to guard the privacy of patient data. They are subject to substantial penalties for each instance in which patient data are accessed by anyone other than a person who has a "need to know." Yet, as is evident from violations that are reported both in healthcare and in other sectors of the economy, securing data with absolute assurance that security will not be violated is challenging. In healthcare, there is a wide diversity of human beings, both inside the

Table 11.3 Healthcare IT Standards Organizations

Global Standards Organizations		
Acronym	**Organization**	**Standard**
ISO	International Organization for Standardization	Healthcare and others
IEC	International Electrical Commission	Computer
ITU	International Telecommunication Union	Telecommunications
HL7	Health Level 7	HER, messaging, and communication
UN/EDIFACT	UN/EDI Finance, Administration, Commerce and Transportation	EDI
UN/CEPFACT	UN Center for Electronic FACT and OASIS	XML and ebXML
DICOM	Digitized Image Communication in Medicine	Medical imaging
IEEE	Institute of Electrical and Electronic Engineers	Network and device communication
CEN	Committee for European Normalisation	ISO
OMG	Object Management Group	UML, CORBA
WHO	World Health Organization	Classification of diseases
IHTSDO	International Health Terminology Standards Development Organization	SNOMED-CT
LOINC	Logical Object Identifiers Nomenclatures Codes	Laboratory
IHE	Integrating the Healthcare Enterprise	Interoperable profiles
CCHIT	Commission on Certification of Health Information Technology	

Source: Kwak, Y.S. Presentation at HIMSS 2008 Annual Conference & Exhibition.

provider organization and outside, who with their own ID and password can access patient data. The organization is reliant on technology security, education, trust, and policies that carry heavy penalties for employees or other stakeholders who violate that trust. For providers, patient information privacy violations can incur civil penalties of up to $25,000, of $50,000 and imprisonment of one year for criminal violations, and if the violation is made under false pretenses the penalty may be up to $100,000 and imprisonment for five years. If the violation is made with intent to sell, transfer, or use individually identifiable information for commercial advantage, personal gain, or malicious hare, the penalty may be up to $250,000 and 10 years in prison.

■ Data sharing: While the healthcare industry, providers and vendors, work through the challenges of designing and developing data sharing networks, the human element in the sharing of data is yet another challenge to the implementation of the EHR. There is reluctance among providers, hospitals, and physicians alike to share what they have viewed as proprietary data with other providers. They are concerned about how the data will be used, how they might be seen in comparison to other providers, and even whether patients and market share will dwindle.

■ ROI: While it is commonly acknowledged that investments in healthcare IT are critical to fundamental changes in healthcare to improve quality and safety and to improve operational effectiveness and gain efficiencies, return on investment continues to be elusive. "The impact and expectation of cost-justifying patient safety IT initiatives using a traditional ROI must evolve to focus beyond the financial benefit. It must encompass overall patient safety, patient satisfaction, and employee and physician satisfaction benefit categories" (24).

In other words, all of healthcare IT must be looked at and measured more broadly than just on the direct dollar impact. It must be measured on clinical improvements as documented by quality measures (measures made possible by the very IT systems on which ROI is being analyzed), by reductions in medical errors, by improvements in processes, by staff, physician, and patient satisfaction, by improved strategic decision making, by improved communications and other factors, in addition to financial performance, that are all key to the future of the organization.

11.12 Summary

The future of healthcare is tied to its ongoing research and the IT infrastructure that is key to its future, efficiency, effectiveness, and quality initiatives to protect the safety of patients while in hospitals. The potential for genomics to dramatically change the way in which medical care is delivered is awesome — the development of PHC can revolutionize medical care in the capability it has to deliver solutions to health problems that are designed for the individual's genetic structure. However, the ability to take advantage of this research and to get it to the clinical setting is dependent upon the full implementation of the EHR. While the United States is making incredible investments in genomics and healthcare IT, the future can only be shaped by the will to make the results available to all and by the readiness to accept a new way of looking at medicine and at each person's responsibility and potential to control and manage his or her own health.

References

1. J. A. DiMasi, R. W. Hansen, and H. G. Grabowski, 2003. "The price of innovation: New estimates of drug development costs." *Journal of Health Economics*, 22, 151–185.
2. Food and Drug Administration (FDA), 2008. "The New Drug Development Process: Steps from Test Tube to New Drug Application Review." Accessed January 2009. Available at: http://www.fda.gov/CDER/HANDBOOK/DEVELOP.HTM
3. "Human Genome Project Information," 2008. Accessed December 2008. Available at: http://www.ornl.gov/sci/techresources/Human_Genome/medicine/pharma.shtml
4. J. Carpenter, M. Farrell, R. Franco, L. Huang, and G. Kirunda, 2007. "Research and Genomics." A research paper prepared to meet the requirements of graduate work in the Masters in Medical Informatics Program, Northwestern University, Chicago, IL.
5. National Institute of General Medical Sciences, 2006.
6. H. Moses, E. R. Dorsey, D. H. M. Matheson, and S. O. Their, 2005. "Financial Anatomy of Biomedical Research." *Journal of the American Medical Assoication* 294:1333–1342.
7. Genetic Information Nondiscrimination Act: 2007–2008. Web Accessed November 2008. Available at: http://www.genome.gov/24519851
8. National Human Genome Research Institute, 2007. Accessed October 2008. Available at: http://www.fda.gov/cder/genomics/
9. National Institute of Health (NIH), National Human Genome Research Institute, 2009. "Genetic Information Nondiscrimination Act: 2007–2008." Accessed January 2009. Available at: http://www.genome.gov/24519851
10. E. Abrahams, G. S. Ginsburg, and M. Silver, 2005. "The personalized medicine coalition: Goals and strategies." *American Journal of Pharmacogenomics*, 5(6):345–355.
11. American Hospital Association (AHA), 2005. "Forward momentum: Hospital use of information technology." Accessed October 2008. Available at: http://www.aha.org/aha/content/2005/pdf/FINALNonEmbITSurvey105.pdf
12. S. Fox. PEW Internet and American Life Project. "Online Health Search 2006." October 2006. Accessed October 2008. Available at: http://www.perinternet.org/pdfs/PIP_Online_Health_2006.pdf

13. Agency for Healthcare Research and Quality (AHRQ), 2008. "Health Information Technology." Accessed October 2008. Available at: http://healthit.ahrq.gov.
14. National Conference of State Legislatures Forum for State Health Policy Leadership, 2008. "Frequently Asked Questions." Accessed October 2008. Available at: http://www.ncsl.org/pring/health/forum/HIT_FAQ.pdf
15. Walker, J., Pan, E., Johnston, D., Adler-Milstein, J., Bates, D., Middleton, B., January 2005. "The Value of Health Care Information Exchange and Interoperability." *Health Affairs*. Available at: http://healthaff.highwire.org/cgi/reprint/htlhaff/w5.10v1.pdf
16. Health Information and Management Systems Society (HIMSS), 2008. "Electronic Health Record." Accessed November 2008. Available at: http://www.himss.org/ASP/topics_ehr.asp
17. Health Information and Management Systems Society, HIMSS Analytics (HIMMS), 2007. "Essentials of the US Hospital IT Market 2007." Accessed October 2008. Available at: http://www.himssanalytics.org/docs/e07_chapter-intro.pdf
18. eHealth Initiative, Foundation for eHealth Initiative, 2008. "2008 Survey Report." Accessed October 2008. Available at: http://ehealthinitiative.org/HIESurvey/2008 StateOfTheField.mspx
19. Markle Foundation Connecting for Health, a Public-Private Collaborative, 2003. The Personal Health Working Group Final Report, July 1, 2003. Accessed October 2008. Available at: http://www.marklefoundation.org
20. Center for Drug Evaluation and Research, 2006. Accessed October 2008. Available at: http://www.fda.gov/cder/
21. National Institute of Standards and Technology (NIST), 2008. Rhodes, Tom. "Health Care Standards Landscape." Accessed October 2008. Available at: http://www.itl.nist.gov/div897/docs/hc_roadmap.html
22. Health Information and Management Systems Society (HIMMS), 2008. "Journal: Who's Counting Now? ROI for Patient Safety IT Initiatives" Accessed October 2008. Available at: http://www.himss.org/ASP/issuesdetail.asp?faid=30&ContentID=38499&SubTypeName=Journal

Index